I0415419

ANTI INFLAMMATORY DIET FOR BEGINNERS

A 3-weeks anti-inflammatory diet plan for beginners with easy recipes to fight inflammation and restore general health

Hanna Greenberg

The information provided herein is stated to be truthful and consistent, in that any liability, in terms of inattention or otherwise, by any usage or abuse of any policies, processes, or directions contained within is the solitary and utter responsibility of the recipient reader. Under no circumstances will any legal responsibility or blame be held against the publisher for any reparation, damages, or monetary loss due to the information herein, either directly or indirectly.

Respective authors own all copyrights not held by the publisher.

The information herein is offered for informational purposes solely, and is universal as so. The presentation of the information is without contract or any type of guarantee assurance.

The trademarks that are used are without any consent, and the publication of the trademark is without permission or backing by the trademark owner. All trademarks and brands within this book are for clarifying purposes only and are the owned by the owners themselves, not affiliated with this document.

Table of contents

Hanna Greenberg

INTRODUCTION

Fitness and-Health: "Taking care of one's health has dependably been a significant concern for people. Throughout the previous 150 years or something like that, the Western world has come to understand that people should deal with their health in a balanced and scientific way. Diet has been the most usable and practical region of concern the extent that health care is concerned.

Naturally, diet programs have increased colossal significance, and an ever-increasing number of people are getting to be health aware, however, diet cognizant too. The majority of the people are concerned about the fundamental part of a diet program - they need to lose weight.

Although weight loss remains the primary concern, diet programs are additionally followed for weight gain, sugar control, a decrease of body hair, and different contemplations. One may bring up issues in regards to the very idea of diet programs, yet one ought to always remember that these programs are bound to shift from person to person.

Likewise, these programs can be set for a specific person directly after the person experiences a fast registration, and his therapeutic history is considered. The best possible importance of diet, in any case, is to follow a specific routine of sustenance admission relying upon one's body condition. It can likewise be said that diets give the premise of figuring out how to eat appropriately.

If you have sufficient energy and devotion to follow such diet programs, you are bound to get good outcomes. Many diet programs (counting on the web diet programs) are very trendy nowadays, offering a ton of data on nourishment and fitness and giving a solid base with the goal that you can figure out how to eat more healthily.

There are numerous legends that people accept to be realities. Like you can't eat past 8 o'clock around evening time. You can, however, just if you accomplish something after you eat. Numerous people feel that carbs make them put on weight. Although they do, there are two are things they need to forget about and looking for in concerns to how they're putting on weight.

Most importantly if you need to lose weight, you need to roll out little improvements everyday and create new propensities for yourself. Does that mean you need to quit eating pastries? No, it doesn't. There are reasons why surrendering your preferred sustenances really can hurt your weight loss efforts and how to healthfully adjust what's right for you and what you wish was good for you.

There are likewise practices that you can accomplish for nothing, every day, for as meager as a couple of minutes to enable you to consume your weight.

However, the important thing is to realize the difference between weight loss and fat loss! Because you are getting in shape does not mean you are losing fat. You could be losing water weight from a low-carb diet, fasting, low-calorie diet, or from attempting a craze diet or taking "enchantment" pills. How does this affect your body, and how would you lose fat? These are things you need to know to spare yourself time, cash, and potential health perils.

CHAPTER ONE

The Anti-Inflammatory Diet

Chronic inflammation is a type of inflammation that silently assaults the body causing disease and degeneration, and is otherwise called "silent inflammation." As the connection between silent inflammation and a large group of diseases becomes more evident, the case for dietary and lifestyle changes that can battle inflammation has become stronger. While it was always referred to that some conditions, for example, joint pain and acne were a result of acute inflammation in the body, there is mounting evidence that silent inflammation assumes a role in heart disease, Alzheimer's, diabetes and some cancers, just as in the maturing process. Chronic inflammation can be present undetected in your body for quite a long time until it manifests in disease.

Silent inflammation has been associated with the buildup of cholesterol deposits in the arteries, which can lead to heart disease. Along these lines, the danger of Alzheimer's disease increases with inflammation of mind tissue, as this results in the buildup of amyloid plaque deposits in the cerebrum. Having type 2 diabetes, or eating sugary foods contributes to silent inflammation in the body as a result of elevated glucose and insulin levels. Recent studies have likewise confirmed the connection between inflammation and several types of cancers. Making the necessary lifestyle changes to battle inflammation can protect you from its devastating effects.

There are molecules in the body called prostaglandins, which assume a significant role in inflammation. It has been found out that of the three primary types of prostaglandins, two of them (PG-E1 and PG-E3) have an anti-inflammatory effect, while the third type (PG-E2) promotes inflammation. When there is an imbalance in the body between these prostaglandins, inflammation can result. Prostaglandins are made in the body from essential unsaturated fats. You can help your body in making anti-Inflammatory prostaglandins by eating vegetables, nuts, grains, and seeds, for example, sesame and sunflower seeds. Then again, foods that cause a spike in insulin levels, for example, sugary foods, or foods with a high Glycemic load promote the generation of PG-E2 and increase inflammation.

A run of the mill anti-inflammatory diet focuses on battling inflammation through the utilization of foods that lower insulin levels. To actively reduce inflammation, you ought to, therefore, eat foods that have a low Glycemic load, for example, whole grains, vegetables, and lentils, and consume healthy fats, for example, nuts, seeds, fish, extra virgin olive oil and fish. Spices, for example, turmeric, ginger, and hot peppers additionally reduce inflammation. At the same time, you additionally need to reduce utilization of foods that are star inflammatory, for example, red meat, egg yolks, and shellfish. Sugar is a critical guilty party in inflammation, and therefore, you should likewise reduce sugary foods. Inflammation can similarly be reduced by taking supplements, for example, fish oils which are high in Omega 3 unsaturated fats.

Anti inflammatory diet

The Benefits of an Anti-Inflammatory Diet

Inflammation is rapidly turning into the following substantial medical discovery. People suffering from stoutness have inflammation issues. Diabetes, joint pain, and asthma are altogether connected with inflammation in the body. Also, the connection to certain heart conditions and malignant growths. Diminishing the inflammation in your body with an anti-inflammation diet can make a quick change how you feel, also the long-haul impacts of the dietary change on health and prosperity.

The initial step to embracing an anti-inflammatory diet is to comprehend the impacts of foods on the body. Food gives supplements and nutrients the body needs to endure. The idea of eating to live not living to eat is a tremendous push for the weight reduction network, yet this idea ought not merely to be pursued when expecting to shed a couple of pounds. Certain foods have high groupings of anti-oxidants and natural anti-inflammatory supplements that may reduce the impact of inflammation on the body. It is these foods that foundation the anti-inflammatory diet.

The Role of Omega 3 and Other Fatty Acids

Fatty acids are available in many foods that contain oil. The best natural source is fish like salmon and sardines. In any case, Omega 6 fatty acids are pervasive in western diets over Omega 3s. This is because essential eaten foods like chicken, turkey, eggs, nuts, and vegetable oils are wealthy in Omega 6 fatty acids. What people don't understand, be that as it may, is that these fatty acids should be offset with Omega 3s for ideal health and anti-inflammatory activity. Most western diets incorporate multiple times more Omega 6s than Omega 3s. A few diets include as much as numerous times more. The ideal proportion is 4 sections Omega 6 to each 1 section Omega 3.

Expanding Omega 3 fatty acids in the diet can reduce inflammation in the body and hence reduce the impact of this condition on health and general prosperity. Foods wealthy in Omega 3s incorporate fish oil, kiwi, dark raspberry, and different nuts. The most readily accessible source of Omega 3s is flaxseeds.

Numerous people misstep fish oils for the best source, yet flaxseed oils will, in general, have the most readily available Omega 3s that make retention in the body more unaffected. Flaxseed oils contain about 55% ALA (alpha-linolenic acid) which is an Omega 3 fatty acid.

Fatty Meats Be Gone

Another necessary change to reduce inflammation in the body is the decrease in fatty meats. Red meat is the most noticeably terrible of all meats for people suffering from inflammation. Picking a less fatty cut or a less greasy option is a decent choice. Buffalo and venison are two choices that will, in general, contain less fat. Grass bolstered dairy animals additionally have less inflammatory qualities on the body. Fish, lean chicken, turkey, soybeans, tofu, and soy milk are, for the most part, thin decisions for diminishing inflammation. A portion of these meats will, in general, be higher in Omega 6s. To battle the fatty acid irregularity that might expand inflammation, take a stab at cooking these meats in olive oil or adding flaxseed oil to the last dish to help Omega 3s.

The Danger of Processed Foods

The most noticeably terrible food to eat when suffering from inflammation is a handled sugar. These foods offer next to no health benefit and ought to be supplanted with entire grain choices. All flour is wheat-based. However, handled flour is deprived of the healthy grain wholeness and faded. What is left are empty calories sure to swell the body much more. Essentially supplanting white bread with whole-grain bread and white flour with whole wheat flour that is unbleached can have a major effect on how your body responds to your diet.

The Biggest Struggles of an Anti-Inflammatory Diet

Everybody needs to feel good and live in better health. One of the most straightforward approaches to accomplish that is by changing from a conventional western diet to an anti-inflammatory diet. Rolling out the improvement is simple, however much like a diet plan, staying with the food changes and watching what you eat can be difficult.

Fast Food and Your Inflammation

Fast food is a tremendous deterrent to the anti-inflammatory diet. Foods that are high in fat will in general increment inflammatory substances in the body for three to four hours after the feast. If a similar number of calories eaten in one fast-food sitting were eaten as new natural products, vegetables, and lean meats, this impact would not happen. Free radicals, cell executioners that compound inflammation issues, can likewise be expanded by 175% in the wake of eating fast food.

The Alternative - The best alternative to fast food is a substitution, anti-inflammatory diet. Take the Big Mac from McDonald's into thought. This sandwich can be produced using lean ground turkey and an entire grain bun. The "extraordinary" sauce can be stirred up with lower starch ketchup, olive oil mayonnaise, and sugar-free relish. The outcome is a delicious alternative with a significantly lower fat check.

Red Meat, Milk and Your Inflammation

Science has long battled to interface red meat with specific types of malignant growth. Much to their dismay, the examination would prompt a connection between this healthy supper protein and inflammation. Scientists accept the body responds to certain substance parts of red meat and milk defensively. If the body agrees with these are outside substances, the insusceptible framework will kick in, and inflammation happens. Envision eating red meat once every day and drinking a few glasses of milk. The body would live in a condition of consistent or constant inflammation, which could cause health issues after some time.

The Alternative - Lean poultry, beef, and fish are all piece of a healthy diet. Meat is an incredible source of iron, so killing it's anything but a need. Be that as it may, choosing the least fatty of slices is fundamental to great health. The best meats are lean proteins and beans.

Trans Fats and Your Inflammation

A concealed source of body inflammation is trans fatty acid. While numerous individuals realize somewhat about this kind of fat, few comprehend the consequences for the body. Fast food, baked goods, prepackaged dinners, and margarine are regularly great sources of trans fat. In the wake of entering the body, these fats can build the danger of coronary vein illness, insulin opposition, diabetes, and heart disappointment. The expanded risk of stroke because of exceptional high lipid levels is additionally usual. While many foods will profess to be trans-fat-free, that isn't the whole truth. As indicated by naming rules, these foods can contain up to 0.5 grams of trans fats per serving and still imprint the item as "trans-fat-free." These modest quantities will include after some time if the diet is wealthy in prepared foods, margarine, and baked goods.

The Alternative - Natural fats like entire margarine and olive oil have no trans fats. Choosing these instead of hydrogenated oils and margarine is a decent initial step. When it comes to foods cooked in trans-fat, there is no decision, however, to dispose of these from the diet altogether. Numerous individuals embrace an anti-inflammatory diet by preparing their tidbits and cooking "fast food" style dinners at home.

Anti-Inflammatory Diet Plan

A portion of our bodies are as of now ablaze within, and a part of our propensities are equivalent to tossing oil on that fire.

That is the thing that I will disclose today - How to put that fire out, or possibly get it back leveled out.

To recap, inflammation is the body's natural response of endeavoring to secure itself. It means to expel hurtful upgrades, for example, pathogens, harmed cells, and aggravations; this is the initial step of the recuperating procedure.

Inflammation triggers a response from the insusceptible framework. At first, inflammation is useful as it is utilized for insurance, yet a lot of the time inflammation can prompt further inflammation (Chronic), which prompts enormous medical issues.

The five signs to pay unique mind to inflammation are torment, redness, heat, swelling, and loss of capacity!

What causes inflammation in any case?

Interminable contaminations

Weight

Environmental toxins (food, water, and air)

Physiological pressure

Escalated/aerobic exercise

Physical injury

Age

Immune system illness

If you see that in the sections for environmental toxins is food.

In this book, I need to talk about the anti-inflammatory diet.

Each food we eat gets a response from the body.

There are certain foods contained in numerous individuals' diet today, which lead to an expansion in inflammation. You can presumably think about what sorts of foods these are (phony foods, fricasseed foods, processed foods, refined carbs, espresso, liquor).

The anti-inflammatory diet contains many foods, which I have prescribed for different purposes, which help to stop and reduce inflammation.

It is a unique method for improving your wellbeing and recouping from ailment or damage.

Without inflammation to stress over you will be a lot more advantageous and less in danger of getting some exceptionally destructive sicknesses over the long haul.

So, what gives you the anti-inflammation diet?

This diet is comprised of an assortment of healthy foods packed with dietary benefit. There are no processed foods, and everything is healthy and healthy.

So, here are the principle foods which are contained in the anti-inflammation diet:

Inflammation Fighting Fats!

Healthy fats make up an enormous extent of the anti-inflammation diet. Foods with high in Omega-3 fatty acids have been demonstrated to be, so I prescribe eating the same number of these foods to help fight inflammation.

Fish is an excellent source, so stock up on sardines, salmon, herring and anchovies. Other great sources incorporate additional virgin olive oil, coconut oil, avocado oil, and pecans.

Antioxidant-Rich Fruit and Vegetables

Fruit and vegetables are packed loaded with antioxidants and nutrients; a portion of these nutrients are demonstrated to be anti-inflammatory. The absolute best wellsprings of vegetables incorporate onions, spinach, sweet potato, peppers, garlic, broccoli, and other green verdant vegetables.

High fruits and berries to pay unique mind to are blueberries, papaya, pineapple, and strawberries. They are packed with high antioxidant content, which is celebrated on such a diet.

Top-notch Protein

Which proteins you eat are essential. There is a major difference between modest value meats and grass encouraged natural meats. The decent value meats will no doubt be packed with hormones and pesticides, which lead to inflammation, while grass bolstered natural meat will fight inflammation.

Pick your meat astutely and go for the omega-3 packed grass encouraged forms as frequently as possible. Utilize this standard when it comes to eggs too. Steak, fish, eggs and poultry and beans (vegetables).

These three kinds of foods structure the foundation of the anti-inflammation diet.

Likewise, herbs and spices, including ginger, curcumin, turmeric, oregano, and rosemary, contain important substances which reduce inflammation and help to restrain perilous free extreme generation.

Food to Avoid no matter what on an Anti-Inflammation Diet

I have quite recently referenced the foods that can prompt a decrease in inflammation, which will keep you healthy. These foods I'm going to refer to are the foods which cause inflammation, and you should evade these.

It's an exercise in careful control.

Master Inflammatory foods:

- Processed foods

- Inexpensive food and takeaways - southern style foods particularly

- Omega 6 fats - you can discover these in numerous oils like sunflower and soybean oil.

- Bread - most wheat and gluten-containing items

- All trans-fats

- Sugar and flour

- Bacon and frankfurters

- Margarine

Tips to Starting Your Anti-Inflammation Diet

The initial steps, likewise with a lot of good diets, are to start to remove the foods that are keeping you down.

So, if you routinely eat any of the above foods just referenced, then you have to begin to remove them. Eating these sorts of foods on an anti-inflammation diet defeats the motivation behind what you are attempting to do and will demolish your outcomes.

Regardless of whether you don't experience the ill effects of inflammation, however, need to change your eating propensities at that point following this sort of diet will, in any case, be beneficial for you. It will build your wellbeing much and will help with fat misfortune.

The subsequent stages are starting to bring anti-inflammation foods into your diet. Start with including the healthy omega 3 fats. Begin to utilize additional virgin olive oil with your vegetables, coconut oil with your cooking, begin eating with nuts instead of chocolate bars and crisps and begin to eat all the newer fish.

Enhancing with a top-notch fish oil supplement is additionally essential.

Ideally, you as of now eat a lot of fruit and vegetables in your diet, if not then you should begin to include them now.

A great aspect regarding fruit and veg is an assortment.

There are genuinely several different assortments of fruit and vegetables accessible to us, all packed with goodness and Flavor.

Drink green tea - Drinking green tea is demonstrated to have anti-inflammatory advantages. Flavonoids in the tea have anti-inflammatory mixes which have been appeared to reduce the danger of specific sicknesses and infections. Be careful that green tea contains caffeine.

Analysis with herbs and spices - Bring some life to your cooking and begin to blend things up. Numerous individuals when cuisine will include salt, sugar, mayonnaise and other simple alternatives begin to add garlic, ginger, turmeric, cayenne, and different herbs and spices to give your supper some genuine flavor without sacrificing the wellbeing of the dinner.

Cut out foods that cause problems - If you find that you are biased to specific foods or you experience the ill effects of issues in the wake of eating certain foods at that point cut them out totally. Numerous individuals get awful responses from wheat, and gluten-containing foods, so give cutting a shot these foods and check whether you see a difference. Dispose of the foods that you speculate cause problems one by one, and you will before long reveal the guilty party!

CHAPTER TWO

Top Ten Anti Inflammatory Foods to Add to Your Diet for Pain Relief

While more people are looking for conventional homeopathic and standard treatment for arthritis, gout, and numerous other muscle and joint a throbbing painfulness, the most comfortable and most practical home solutions for agony might add a couple of top nourishments to eat to the American diet. Here is a short rundown of anti-inflammatory sustenances for wellbeing.

#1 - Fish, mainly a virus water fish like salmon, trout, or fish, is stacked with anti-inflammatory omega-3 fatty acids. Numerous investigations affirm adding fish (or fish oil) to one's diet will lower inflammation.

Pick your fish cautiously There is much discussion over wild fish versus farm-raised. Wild fish are generally higher in supplements and lower in fat than farm-raised, on account of their diet and the activity they get swimming.

Farm-raised fish, on the normal, have about 20% less protein and 20% more fat than wild got. farmed fish eat a diet of small fish, shrimp and red krill, which is the place the bounty of omega-3 EFAs in their substance begins. They are additionally unfenced, and get plentiful exercise, reducing their fat-content.

Farm-raised fish are encouraged fishmeal pellets, generally made of ground, handled and packed mackerel, anchovies, sardines, and other small fish, which does not contain the high convergences of omega-3s than wild nourishment sources do. To imitate the dark red shading that wild fish have, particularly salmon, most farm-raised fish are encouraged a color alongside their dinner. Since fish farms are small, packed net walled in areas or pens. The fish are encouraged antibiotics to battle illnesses, parasites, and diseases.

There have likewise been reports of high mercury content, both in wild and farmed fish: the wild fish from living in debased waters, and the farmed fish from mercury sullying in their feed. Mercury in fish, for the most part, gathers in the skin, so while eating fish, you should not eat the skin.

#2 - *Extra Virgin Olive is a great source of oleic acid*; an anti-inflammatory oil. Olive oil additionally improves insulin work in this way, lowering glucose. Due to its low smoke point, olive oil isn't useful for profound singing, however, is ideal for more beneficial cooking choices, for example, sauté and braising — Cook with olive oil instead of oils or shortening that are high in undesirable trans-fats.

#3 - Walnuts, Nuts Almonds, cashews, and many different nuts are high in oleic acid, just as omega-3 fatty acids, fiber, protein, and other sound phytochemicals. Since certain nuts are high in fat, make sure to eat them with some restraint.

#4 - Grapes Discovery report that grapes are high in flavonoids, which they accept have anti-inflammatory properties. As indicated by Medical news today "Now, specialists at the Johns Hopkins University School of Medicine have shown that powdered grapes seem to lessen agony and inflammation in a rodent model of arthritis, where rodents' knees are kindled utilizing a chemical infusion." may be drinking wine, as the Europeans know, can lower inflammation also.

#5 - Cherries, particularly tart cherries, are a rich source of antioxidants. Specifically, they contain a lot of anthocyanins, a standout amongst the most dominant antioxidants, which give the cherries their rich, red shading.

An investigation directed by the Agricultural Research Service (ARS) researchers and their college associates recommends that cherries may diminish severe ligament inflammation, just as reducing the danger of other inflammatory conditions, for example, cardiovascular sickness and malignant growth.

#6 - Green Tea Green tea, which is an unfermented tea, contains flavonoids called "catechins." Catechins are incredible antioxidants which are obliterated during the handling and aging procedure that different teas experience. Green tea provides about 27% catechins, rather than oolong (halfway matured) which includes 23%, and dark tea (aged) which contains about 4%. Creature studies have shown that green tea significantly diminished the seriousness of arthritis. As per the National Center for Complementary and Alternative Medicine (NCCAM), green tea influences arthritis by causing changes in arthritis-related resistant reactions.

If you find you have cerebral pains in the wake of devouring teas, you may have a sensitivity, the same number of individuals find. As usual, tune in to your body and see what works.

#7 - Leafy Greens Green verdant vegetables, for example, spinach and kale, are pressed with fiber, antioxidants, and Omega 3s.

Search for naturally developed produce, or make sure to wash altogether to evacuate the chemicals and pesticides that will result in general amass on the leaves.

#8 - Broccoli A compound, 3,3'-diindolylmethane (DIM), found in broccoli and its kissing cousins, cauliflower and Brussels grows, has been shown to battle inflammation and help support the invulnerable framework. These super-veggies likewise contain sulfolane, a phytonutrient that helps liver capacity and builds your body's regular detoxification capacity. Eat them crude (solidified assortments of vegetables lose a lot of health benefits) or steam them to protect the valuable supplements, which can be separated by cooking techniques, for example, boiling or singing.

#9 - Apples and red onions both contain quercetin, a chemical that examination has shown to have anti-inflammatory properties, alongside different antioxidants. Most of the quercetin is in their skins. It's what gives them their rich red shading, so don't strip apples before you eat them. Flush all fresh leafy foods a long time before eating to help dispense with pesticides and manures.

#10 - Water The more crisp, clean water you drink, the better. Your body is comprised of over 70% water, and consistent recharging keeps poisons flushed from your framework, including joints, muscles, and blood.

As of late, with the expanded prevalence of bottled water, there has been heated discussion over tap water versus bottled water. To choose which is better for you, you should realize what the differences are.

There is a bewildering exhibit of decisions in bottled water accessible available today, from spring water, mineral water, well water, to shining water. While some of them originate from usual springs and other perfect sources, over 25% of the bottled water sold originates from metropolitan sources.

That is correct. You might drink tap water!

Astute bundling messages have corralled the crowd attitude of an accommodating, idealistic open!

It's been treated, filtered and purified, at that point bottled and offered to you at a thousand-overlap increment in cost. There are no ebb and flow guidelines that power the bottler to a state where the water originates from, so flawless mountain icy mass liquefy that you thought you were drinking may have in reality originated from a tap in Alaska or New Jersey.

Bottled water is no more beneficial than tap water. Momentum research proposes that it might be increasingly unsafe. BPA's, chemical in the plastic of the bottles themselves, can escape into the water you are drinking. (BPAs are known to cause neurological issues, in addition to other things.)

Notwithstanding the perils of the chemicals in the bottles, there are other natural impressions to consider. Fossil fuels, with their related contamination and nursery gasses, are utilized to create plastic bottles. Delivery water bottles far and wide use up progressively fossil fuels, just as causing carbon contamination of our air and waterways. When almost plastic water bottles are recyclable, over 75% of them end up in landfills, or littering shorelines, lakes, and the sides of the street.

Take a gander at your tap water.

Metropolitan water sources are thoroughly treated and tried by the EPA. EPA guidelines of contaminants are severe, while the FDA guidelines for bottled water are a lot looser. Tap water likewise contains fluoride, to help shield our teeth from rot. In particular, tap water is incredibly wallet cordial! Twenty ounces of water from the kitchen fixture costs pennies, yet twenty ounces of bottled water costs over $1.

If the flavor of the bottled water is the thing that keeps you getting it, consider adding a filter to your tap water at home. There are numerous filters accessible in a gigantic scope of costs, from straightforward pitchers that filter water for around $20, as far as possible up to complex frameworks for your whole house that cost a large number of dollars. Make sure to look at that it doesn't filter the fluoride that your teeth need. If you like the comfort of the convenient bottle, consider putting resources into a reasonable reusable bottle made of a more secure, progressively sturdy plastic, for example, that used to ship water on a bike, or even a glass or metal canteen. Your condition and your wallet will value the exertion.

Eating Anti-Inflammatory Foods

Are there truly diets out there that can reduce inflammation? Do they work? Researchers have discovered that there is a relationship, to some degree, between what we eat and inflammation. They've even identified a few mixes in food that can reduce inflammation and others that advance it. There is still a long way to go about exactly how diet and inflammation cooperate and inquire about, starting at yet, isn't by then where specific foods or gatherings of foods can be singled out as being gainful for people with Arthritis. We are starting to get a clearer picture of how eating the correct way can reduce inflammation.

So, for what reason would we say we are so worried about inflammation? Inflammation is the body's collective resistance to diseases and wounds. When something turns out badly, the body's safe framework gets down to business to arouse the region, which serves to dispose of the trespasser or to mend the injury. Inflammation can cause torment, swelling, redness, and warmth. However, this leaf when the issue is understood. This is a high inflammation.

At that point, we have chronic inflammation, the sort that is comfortable for people with rheumatoid Arthritis (RA), lupus, psoriatic Arthritis, and different kinds of "inflammatory" Arthritis. Chronic inflammation is the sort that won't leave. Every one of the types of Arthritis that are referenced above are a turmoil of the safe framework makes inflammation, and after that doesn't have a clue when to close off. Inflammatory Arthritis, chronic inflammation can have genuine outcomes, lasting incapacity, and tissue harm can be one if it isn't dealt with appropriately. Inflammation has been connected to a full host of other ailments.

Inflammation has been found to add to atherosclerosis, which is when fat develops on the covering of courses, raising the danger of heart assaults. Additionally, high degrees of inflammation proteins have been found in the blood of people with heart disease. Inflammation has additionally been connected to obesity, diabetes, asthma, misery, and significantly Alzheimer disease and malignant growth. Researchers feel that a consistent degree of inflammation in the body, regardless of whether the level is low, can have various negative impacts. Research demonstrates that diet can reduce inflammation; in principle, an inflammation-lowering diet ought to affect a wide scope of health conditions.

Analysts have searched for intimations in the eating habits of our early ancestors to find which foods may profit us the most. They accept those habits are more to our eating habits with how the body procedures and utilizations what we eat and drink. Our ancestor's diet comprised of wild lean meats (venison or pig) and wild plants (verdant green vegetables, natural products, nuts, and berries). There were no oat grains until the agribusiness transformation (around 10,000 years back). There was almost no dairy, and there were no handled or refined foods. Our diets are generally are high in meat, immersed (or awful) fats, and handled foods, and there is almost no activity. Nearly all that we eat is accessible close by or as far away as our PC and the snap of a mouse.

Our diet and lifestyles are way askew with how our bodies are produced using the back to front. While our hereditary make-up has changed next to no from our early beginnings, our diet and lifestyles have changed a lot, and the progressions have deteriorated in the course of the last 50 to 100 years. Our qualities haven't got an opportunity to adjust. We aren't giving our bodies the correct sort of fuel. It's just as we think about our bodies as motors in a stream plane when somewhat they resemble the motor in the absolute first planes. There are a few foods that we are putting into our bodies, mainly because we are eating way a lot of them, that are influencing our health worse.

There are two supplements in our diets that have stood out, are omega-3 fatty acids and omega-6 fatty acids have been a piece of our diets for a large number of years. They are parts in pretty much the majority of our numerous cells and are significant for healthy development and advancement. Both of these acids assume a job in inflammation. In a few examinations, it was discovered that specific sources of omega 3's specifically, help to reduce the inflammation procedure and that omega 6's will raise it.

Presently this is the issue. The average American eats by and large around multiple times more omega 6's than omega 3's. While our in all respects early ancestor's ate omega 6's and omega 3's in equivalent proportion, and it is accepted this is the thing that reasonable their capacity to turn inflammation on and off. The unevenness of omega 3's and omega 6's in our diets is accepted to add to the abundance of inflammation in our bodies.

So, can any anyone explain why we eat such a significant number of omegas 6's presently? Vegetable oils, for example, corn oil, safflower oil, sunflower oil, cottonseed oil, soybean oil, and the items produced using them, for example, margarine, are stacked with omega 6's. Indeed, even vast numbers of the handled nibble foods that are so promptly accessible today are loaded with these oils. Given the best data of the time, was to utilize vegetable oils like those referenced above rather than foods with immersed fats, for example, margarine and fat. It would appear that the results of that appeal may have added to the expanded utilization of omega 6's and along these lines causing an awkwardness of omega 3's and omega 6's.

You can discover omega 6's in other healthy foods, for example, meats and egg yolks. The omega 6 found in beef is the fatty acids that originated from grain-nourished creatures, for instance, bovines, sheep, pigs, and chickens. The more significant part of the meat sold in America is grain sustained not at all like their grass-encouraged cousins who contain less of those fatty acids. Wild game, for example, venison and pig are lower in omega 6's and fat and higher in omega 3's than the meat that originates from the grocery stores where we shop.

You can get omega 3s in both creature and plant food. Our bodies can change over omega 3s from creature sources into anti-inflammatory mixes more effectively than the omega 3s from plant sources. Plant foods contain several other healthful combinations a significant number of which that are anti-inflammatory, so don't limit them all together.

Various foods are high in omega 3s, and that incorporate fatty fish, mainly fish from virus waters. Everybody thinks about salmon however did you realize that you can likewise discover omega 3s in mackerel, anchovies, sardines, herring, striped bass, and bluefish. It's also generally recognized that wild fish are excellent sources of omega 3s over the ranch-raised ones. You can likewise purchase eggs that have been enhanced with omega 3 oils. There are a few incredible sources of omega 3s in plants that are verdant greens (like kale, Swiss chard, and spinach) just as flaxseed, wheat germ, pecans, and their oils.

You can likewise get omega 3s in enhancements (regularly as fish oil); this source has been demonstrated to be advantageous in specific occurrences. You should take with your specialist before you make a fish oil supplement since it can cooperate with certain meds and in particular situations can build the danger of dying. I take a recommended omega 3 supplements because my specialist had disclosed to me that the ones you get in the grocery store or health food store are not untouched, they have different added substances that do nothing to help. Different fats are supporters of obstructed veins, the "terrible" or soaked fats found in meats and high-fat dairy foods. These are called master inflammatory.

There are likewise the Trans fats that are moderately new to the reason for heart disease. These Trans fats can be found in prepared comfort and nibble foods and can be spotted by perusing the marks. They can be identified as halfway hydrogenated oils, frequently soybean oil or cottonseed oil. However, they can likewise happen generally in limited quantities in creature foods. The idea is that they add to the professional inflammatory exercises in our bodies, and the sums we eat today are incredible.

Antioxidants are substances that counteract inflammation-causing "free radicals" from overtaking our bodies. Plant foods, for example, natural products, vegetables (counting beans), nuts, and seeds, convey high measures of antioxidants. Extra-virgin olive oil and pecan oil are generally excellent sources of antioxidants, moreover. These foods have for quite some time been viewed as the nuts and bolts for good health and can be found in products of the soil with bright and lively colors. The more beautiful the plant, the better they are for you, from green vegetables, particularly green ones, to low-starch vegetables, for example, broccoli and cauliflower, to berries, tomatoes, and splendidly hued orange and yellow leafy foods.

I wager you're pondering what this has to do with Arthritis. There has been some exploration on diet and Arthritis, generally concentrating on RA. There was a study that investigated a lot of different examinations on diet and RA and found that diets high in omega 3's had some impact on lessening the indications of RA. There was one more study distributed in 2008, that discovered eating omega 6 fatty acids and omega 3 fatty acids in a proportion of 2 or 3 to

1 (a low balance contrasted with the 15 to 1 proportion in a great many people's diet) diminished the inflammation in people with RA. There was additionally another study that discovered taking omega 3 may likewise allow people to reduce their utilization of no steroidal anti-inflammatory medications (NSAIDs, for example, ibuprofen (Advil, Motrin) and naproxen (Aleve). In any case, these and different examinations don't offer enough proof to demonstrate that there is a specific anti-inflammatory diet that can affect arthritis indications. It doesn't imply that the diets are destructive; it just means that there may come a multi-day when research might most likely demonstrate their advantages. Later on, a diet might be viewed as one of the numerous devices alongside exercise and medication that can be utilized to facilitate the side effects of Arthritis.

We don't need to return totally to the caveman to eat the anti-inflammatory way to profit by the anti-inflammatory diet. Only eating a healthful diet that is prescribed today is spot on the track. Our central technique ought to be to adjust the measure of cutting-edge foods with the foods of sometime in the past, which were wealthy in the inflammation lessening foods. Vitally, we should simply supplant foods wealthy in omega 6 with foods wealthy in omega 3, eliminating how much meat and poultry we eat while eating oily fish several times each week and including more assortments of beautiful products of the soil, and keeping in mind that entire grains were not a piece of our early ancestor's diet, it ought to be incorporated into our own. Make sure that it is whole grains and not refined grains since they contain numerous helpful supplements and inflammation-treating mixes. Specialists have discovered that eating a lot of foods high in sugar and white flour may advance inflammation, although there are additionally studying that should be done regarding the matter.

The measures of information we have on how the body functions and how our ancestors ate is affirming the familiar maxim: "For getting healthy, the kind of food you eat is everything." But there is still more we have to learn before we can endorse anyone anti-inflammatory diet. Our hereditary cosmetics and the seriousness of our health condition will decide the advantages we get from an anti-inflammatory diet, and sadly, there is a question that there will be one diet that fits all of us.

Likewise, what we eat or don't eat is only a little piece of the entire story. We are not as physically dynamic as our ancestors, and physical activity has its very own anti-inflammatory impacts. Our ancestors were additionally much slenderer than we are, and body fat is active tissue that can make inflammatory creating mixes.

Anti-inflammatory eating is a way of choosing foods that are more tuned in to what the body immensely. We can accomplish a progressively adjusted diet by returning to our underlying foundations. If you take a gander at the diet of the people of the Bible, you will find that they, similar to our caveman ancestors, were increasingly dynamic and their diets comprised of many same things from our caveman ancestors. They additionally had no real option except to walk wherever they needed to go. There was no such thing as autos or trucks. While we have it simpler today, our health has experienced enormously it.

Eat Your Anti-Inflammatory Fruits and Veggies!

Fruits and vegetables are indispensable segments to the anti-inflammatory lifestyle. Eating bountiful measures of the correct types of these disease-battling foods will enable you to improve your health, feel much improved, look better, and have more energy! Incalculable investigations have indicated eating fruits and vegetables diminishes your danger of heart disease, different malignant growths, diabetes, and various other incessant diseases. Your initial step is to start adding non-boring vegetables to your dinners in enormous quantities. Since 4 cups of verdant green vegetables, for example, spinach contains around 30 calories, putting on unhealthy load from these sources isn't an issue! The main vegetables to be for the most part maintained a strategic distance from are bland tubers, for example, potatoes, sweet potatoes, and yams, as these are high glycemic foods that can cause huge spikes in blood sugar. Nonetheless, if you are a competitor preparing for an occasion or inherently captivating in regular overwhelming activity, at that point, these foods can be added to improve your exhibition.

Specific types of fruits are excellent sources of energy over others. Glycemic index and glycemic load are two ideas that have been advanced over the most recent quite a long while and are essential to understanding what foods you ought to eat. The glycemic index estimates how fast specific nourishment triggers a rise in blood sugar. The higher the measure of glucose or fructose in sustenance, the fast it separates and causes an increase in blood sugar and insulin levels. Grains and starches are long chains of glucose held together via carbon bonds. Therefore, they divide all-around rapidly and quickly enter the blood, causing spikes in blood sugar and insulin. Fruits and vegetables, then again, are somewhere in the range of 30 and 70 percent fructose, another type of sugar. Fructose changes overall around gradually to glucose in the liver, so it causes a lot of littler insulin reaction. The higher fiber found in fruits and vegetables likewise acts to hinder the passageway of fructose into the bloodstream further. The total glycemic load of a feast is additionally essential. If high glycemic sustenance, for example, a banana is overcome with low glycemic nourishment, for example, a chicken bosom, the impact on insulin levels will be significantly less extreme than if the banana was eaten alone.

Presently you can perceive any reason why eating a potato or bit of bread, which are 100 percent glucose, causes a more unusual insulin spike than pure table sugar, which is half glucose and half fructose. This is the reason the idea of glycemic load is significantly progressively vital because it considers not just the rate at which sustenance enters the bloodstream. However, the measure of calories it contains. This is important because a few foods have an extremely high absolute glycemic index, however, don't include numerous calories, so their glycemic load is generally low. For instance, a bagel and a serving of watermelon both have a glycemic index of 72, while the glycemic load of the organic product is an unimportant 4 contrasted with 25 for the bagel! The higher the glycemic load of your diet, the more insulin your body is delivering. An examination at Harvard Medical School found the more senior the glycemic load of your diet; the more probable you are to create weight, heart disease, and diabetes. This is an unbelievably talented idea that must be viewed as when choosing what foods to eat.

The extraordinary thing about the anti-inflammatory technique for eating we encourage our patients usually is low glycemic. It should not shock anyone that eating the foods we were intended to eat results in a healthy insulin reaction, not the jolting high points and low points in temperament, energy, and general health that eating a professional inflammatory diet can cause. For instance, an individual who is overweight with Type II diabetes will have altogether different needs, even concerning the type of fruits and vegetables they are eating, then an aggressive tri-competitor consuming a considerable number of calories daily. It can't be underlined enough that this program is specific to your needs, not a one-estimate fits-all methodology.

In the Resources area of your manual, we have included tables with the glycemic index and load of many healthy foods just as plans utilizing low glycemic foods.

Foods that Promote Inflammation

"The more extreme the pain or ailment, the more serious will be the essential changes. These may include getting out from under negative behavior patterns, or procuring some new and better ones." - Peter McWilliams

You are not powerless in your battle against inflammation! Your diet assumes an exceptional job in initiating or stifling a protein considered cytokines that causes inflammation. I must pressure this as much as possible. For that and different reasons that will be examined in no time, I might want you to begin thinking regarding: "Is what I'm gulping making me more beneficial or more wiped out?" There is close to nothing if any unbiased ground. It is as though everything that you swallow is sending a sign to your immune system to either cause more inflammation or less.

Coming up next are gatherings of foods that you ought to keep away from because they send a sign to your body to produce increasingly inflammatory cytokines. They are likewise lethal to your body in various ways, contaminating the interior landscape of the body and advancing inflammation.

Most Meat, Except Oily Fish

We regularly hear the expression "everything with some restraint." Meat, particularly red meat, is a particular case to this standard. Indeed, even what most would consider a "moderate" measure of red meat can produce a terrible number of cytokines and expedite autoimmune symptoms.

For a few, the "low-carb fever" has implied an increase in meat utilization. If eating the low-carb way means that you are eating a great deal of meat, you are aggravating your autoimmune condition. Protein from meat raises the levels of the toxin's uric corrosive and urea in the blood. The body siphons over the top measures of water into the kidneys to help flush out these toxins. The aftereffect of a giant creature-based protein diet is exceptionally speedy water "weight loss." The drawback of this "weight loss" is that it causes the body to lose essential minerals. Mineral insufficiencies cause autoimmunity. A superior protein decision originates from vegetable-based proteins. These proteins improve mineral maintenance in the body.

One specialist includes reported that inside about fourteen days of his lupus patients not eating meat, most indicated significant improvement in their skin sores.

The Swank Diet calls for surrendering red meat for one year. At that point, after the first year, permitting yourself four ounces of red meat every week. This diet has made a significant improvement in the lives of people with Multiple Sclerosis concentrated more than 150 of his patients with M.S. for a thirty-four-year timeframe. The individuals who pursued the diet kicked the bucket at the rate of 5%, while patients not following his diet had a demise rate of about 85% during a similar timeframe.

Be that as it may, reducing meat admission isn't just about living longer; it is tied in with living admirably! This suggestion is for everybody, not merely those whose gathering of autoimmune symptoms are called lupus or M.S. Regardless of where in your body cytokines assemble or what they are assaulting, eating red meat will increase their numbers. How meat is prepared additionally has any effect. Charbroiled and flame-broiled meats of any sort are much more awful for you and ought to be kept away from.

Fish is the exemption to the meat rule. Fish does not raise cytokine levels. It reduces them. The issue is that a lot of our fish is contaminated with poisonous mercury. Except if you are confident that your fish source is sans mercury, you should confine your fish admission to one serving for every week and use fish oil supplements. A few people will even be delicate to one contaminated serving of fish. Check your nearby wellbeing food stores for fish cultivated in "without mercury" tried water. Moreover, salmon is a fish that is promptly accessible and to the least extent liable to be mercury contaminated.

Egg Yolks

Egg yolks and dairy products are high in arachidonic corrosive. This is a similar substance that makes meats so inflammatory. If you eat eggs, you should bite the whites. On a food mark, eggs can be recorded as egg whites, globulin, ovamucin, or vitellin.

Dairy Products

"...countries with the most astounding dairy utilization, for example, the United States and Sweden, because of their high creature protein diets, have the most astounding rates of osteoporosis, a disease including the debilitating and potential breaking of bones."

Research distributed in the Lancet Medical Journal depicted a little gathering of patients with Chronic Fatigue Syndrome (CFS) in Norway. For four years, they encountered generous improvement by barring milk and wheat from their diets. Reintroducing these foods into their diets caused a significant ascent in the patients' cytokine levels alongside an increase in pain.

Other than expanding cytokines, milk further aggravates asthma because of its casein content. When the protein of another creature is brought into the human body, the immune system reacts with an unfavorably susceptible response. Casein is a milk protein. Eating casein causes your body to produce histamines, which result in overabundance bodily fluid production.

Those with CFS and asthma are not the only one in their affectability to milk. As indicated by the New England Journal of Medicine, July

30, 1992, examines propose that a specific milk protein is in charge of the beginning of diabetes because patients produce antibodies to cow milk proteins.

Milk's indecencies are many. As weird as it might sound, the absorption of milk proteins can make an addictive substance that demonstrations like endorphins, our very own opiates. The equivalent can be valid for gluten and wheat. These endorphins can disturb mind science and cause addiction.

I am grieved. However, this must be stated: Last year, the average liter of milk in America contained 323 million discharge cells. Wiped out and tainted dairy animals have cell checks over 200 million. An examination of 323 million isn't even sound by dairy industry models. Drinking discharge is an ill-conceived notion for anybody. It is a horrendous thought for somebody with an inclination towards immune brokenness.

Gluten

Gluten is a segment of grains, for example, wheat, oats, grain, and rye. Other than being inflammatory, specialists have reported a higher than the average number of people with the autoimmune issue are sensitive to gluten. They recommend total shirking for at any rate one month to check whether advantages will happen.

Studies have additionally demonstrated that wheat and corn can irritate patients with Rheumatoid Arthritis and raise cytokine production in the colon and rectum of those with celiac disease.

Corn, Corn Oil, Corn Syrup (Fructose)

Corn, other than advancing cytokines, has been known as the leading cause of perpetual food addiction in this century. To give you a thought of how unusual the habit can be, all cigarettes made in the U.S. since World War I have contained included sugars, generally from corn. Do you think the cigarette organizations picked corn syrup for the incredible taste it adds to their products?

Corn syrup (fructose) is modest and twice as sweet as a natural sweetener. In 1994, the average individual ate 83 pounds of fructose. Corn syrup causes an increase in blood lactic corrosive, particularly in people with diabetes. Fructose from corn syrup restrains copper digestion and diminishes mineral accessibility, two factors in autoimmunity. Fructose likewise separates into a substance that debilitates your body's natural calming atoms. The body does not utilize fructose equivalent to different sugars. Fructose changes over to fat more than some other sugar. Corn fructose surely isn't the diabetic-accommodating and innocuous sugar substitute that it is publicized to be.

Studies have demonstrated that corn can irritate patients with Rheumatoid Arthritis (R.A.) and the National Fibromyalgia Association (NFA) proposes corn ought to be kept away from because it can aggravate Fibromyalgia.

Keep in mind that if corn products can increase cytokine levels in those with R.A. and Fibromyalgia, it can increase cytokine levels for anybody.

Sugar

Americans are eating a normal of 153 pounds of sugar a year. Refined white sugar makes

It progressively difficult for your body to retain nutrients and minerals, a noteworthy supporter of the cause of autoimmunity. Sugar additionally stifles immune capacity, leaving us open to disease. Only eight tablespoons of sugar, which is equal to the sugar in under one 12-ounce jar of soft drink, can reduce the capacity of your immune system to eliminate germs by up to 40%.

Like salt, sugar is drying out to the body. Parchedness increases histamine, which can

Compound asthma and some other autoimmune disease because histamine increases cytokine production. As suggested by the National Fibromyalgia Association (NFA), sugars ought to be maintained a strategic distance from because they can intensify the condition. Sugar sustains Lyme-causing microorganisms and Candida yeast, the significance of which will be talked about later. Eating sugar likewise causes an insulin flood, which adds to constant inflammation.

Nectar is sugar. It might be "all-natural", yet it is still sugar. It is higher in calories than table sugar and can be contaminated by pesticides. Devouring "all-natural" scrumptious tasting pesticides isn't what you need to do.

A decent non-poisonous substitute for sugar is the dietary enhancement stevia. A considerable number of people has utilized stevia without reported reactions. In Japan, improved stevia products speak to 41% of the piece of the pie of sweet substances devoured.

South Americans use it as sugar and furthermore for medicinal purposes. This herb is somewhere in the range of 30 to multiple times better than sugar. Stevia does not influence the blood sugar levels of general diabetics. Stevia likewise does not bolster parasite in the digestion tracts as sugars do.

Stevia has a solid, sweet flavor that can overpower a formula, so it ought to be utilized sparingly. Because you use such a limited quantity at any given moment, plans must be balanced for the absence of mass. Stevia can regularly be obtained with accommodating inulin added to it for celebration. Additionally, cakes and treats improved with stevia don't want dark-colored as much as their sugar-improved partners.

Flour/Processed Foods

For you straightforward starch darlings (addicts), the following sentence will be a standout amongst the most painful ones in the book. If you need to dispose of cytokine inflammation, you should surrender processed foods and lousy nourishments. They will, in general, be brimming with all that you shouldn't eat. This rundown incorporates most breakfast grains, biscuits, bread, saltines, treats, and doughnuts.

White flour contains alloxan, which is the chemical used to make flour look spotless and white. Alloxan obliterates the insulin-delivering beta cells of the pancreas. It does as such by starting free extreme harm to the DNA in the pancreas. Specialists accept that a few people have powerless safeguards to free radicals in these beta cells. Alloxan is potent to the point that specialists who study diabetes use it to offer diabetes to lab creatures. While not every person who eats white bread and processed foods will get diabetes, the association is clear: Alloxan causes diabetes in those hereditarily defenseless to the disease.

The Nightshade Family

Vegetables in the nightshade family incorporate white potatoes, tomatoes, all peppers, fruits, tobacco, and eggplants. Research demonstrates that these vegetables produce pain and inflammation in arthritis patients and aggravate Fibromyalgia, as indicated by the National Fibromyalgia Association (NFA). Notwithstanding, not every person will be touchy to nightshade foods. The best way to know without a doubt is to stay away from them for a time of weeks at that point reintroduce them into your diet.

Everybody ought to keep away from tobacco, which is a dangerous individual from the nightshade family, forever.

Coffee

In spite of being inflammatory, coffee has had its medicinal purposes. My very own progenitors utilized it to treat asthma. I have companions outside, who are as yet subordinate upon coffee to treat asthma. Certain caffeine-type chemicals in coffee have been demonstrated viable at animating bronchial widening in people determined to have specific sorts of asthma. Some cutting-edge asthma meds are even made from chemicals in the caffeine family.

For those utilizing coffee as a natural asthma drug, you should remember that caffeine is a harmful chemical. Its motivation in vegetation is to go about like a bug spray. In people, caffeine stifles the substances required for memory making. It additionally raises both blood sugar and insulin levels, causing cytokine production and severe diabetes.

Mostly drinking decaffeinated coffee isn't the appropriate response either. Ladies who drink more than one cup multi-day of decaffeinated coffee are considered at a lot higher danger of creating rheumatoid arthritis. The hypothesis is that chemically decaffeinated products are causing an increased threat of autoimmunity. If you are to drink decaffeinated coffee in any case, make sure that it utilizes a non-chemical based decaffeinating technique and that the coffee was naturally developed. The individuals who don't drink natural coffee, are presented to too many human-made pesticides.

Alcohol

The wine business has America persuaded that a glass or two dailies is useful for your heart. In any case, a great deal study has done, which demonstrate that to get those heart-solid advantages, you would need to expend enough wine to be declared lawfully alcoholic. Grape juice is a more advantageous option. Dr. Folt's study likewise discovered that lone ten to twelve ounces of purple grape juice was related with lower blood thickening, hence a lower danger of coronary illness than guaranteed by red wine.

Other than being expert inflammatory and addictive, liquor separates to a toxin in the body called aldehyde. Toxins are risky chemicals that the liver does not perceive as valuable. Toxins assault and crush cells and draw in germs. Aldehyde gathers in the cerebrum, spinal rope, joints, muscles, and tissues, where it causes muscle shortcoming, bothering, and pain.

Anti-Inflammatory Foods to Add to Your Diet

I'm not catching inflammation's meaning? It's anything but an infection, although infection can cause inflammation. In reality, inflammation is the body's very own defense

67

attempt to remove destructive improvements, for example, aggravations, damaged cells, etc. This is when inflammation is attempting its healing process.

Inflammation is the first sign when something hurtful or disturbing is affecting pieces of our body. Everyone's body has an immune system, and inflammation is a piece of that. Inflammation is additionally a localized physical condition that results as a reaction to damage or infection, making portions of the body swollen, reddened, painful, and hot. Internal inflammation can happen due to the eating of processed foods, fats, and sugars.

High levels of inflammation can cause several health complexities, for example, arthritis, joint pain, damage to blood vessels, among others. To battle this, it is essential you eat anti-inflammatory foods. kind foods are readily available to add to your diet to control inflammation. These are some of the foods and suggestions to help and keep destructive inflammation under control:

Whole Grains

Whole grains, it is better you consume your grains as whole grains and not refined or pasta. Research has demonstrated that whole grains contain a high amount of fiber, which reduces the inflammatory marker in the blood known as C-reactive protein.

Dark Leafy Greens

Dark leafy vegetables, for example, spinach and kale have high concentrations of vitamin E and minerals, calcium and iron. Studies demonstrate that Nutrient E help in shielding your body from provocative particles known as cytokines. Moreover, dull verdant greens have a high measure of sickness battling phytochemicals.

Fatty Fish

Sleek fish, for example, salmon and fish are foods that are anti-inflammatory as it contains high measures of omega 3 unsaturated fats. The unsaturated fats are known to help joint irritation, so ensure you get a lot of omega 3. Another essential reality about omega 3 is you should get it in your food because the body can't make it inside its system.

Soy

Soybeans contain isoflavones mixes which help the negative impacts of aggravation on joints. In any case, it is excellent you maintain a strategic distance from heavily processed soy items as they may contain added substances and additives. Rather, incorporate soy milk and soybeans into your customary eating routine.

Nuts

Nuts, for example, almonds and pecans are wealthy in vitamin E, calcium, and fiber. Nut is loaded with antioxidants, which can help the body in repairing the damages caused by inflammation.

Berries

Berries are low in fat and calories yet wealthy in antioxidants. Their anti-inflammatory anthocyanins compound in them has numerous great qualities. These helps to prevent you from developing arthritis.

Green Tea

Green tea also has anti-inflammatory flavonoids; this reduces the onset of inflammation and minimizes the danger of certain cancers. It shouldn't be underestimated for some other health benefits. It can reactivate skin cells causing the skin to appear brighter. Drink it regularly and use some honey as a sweetener instead of sugar.

Low Fat Dairy

Low-fat dairy, for example, yogurt contains probiotics which can prevent inflammation. Additionally, dairy foods that are anti-inflammatory, for example, skim milk with high calcium and vitamin D are essential for everyone since separated from having anti-inflammatory properties, they strengthen your bones too.

Ginger and Garlic

Ginger and garlic are anti-inflammatory foods. Both are known to lower body inflammation, control blood sugar levels, and help your body in battling certain infections. Selenium and sulfur in garlic is an essential compound for a healthy immune system. It is likewise one of the top anti-maturing foods you can eat.

Turmeric and Sweet Potato

Turmeric has natural anti-inflammatory compounds called curcumin, which is known to mood killer NF-kappa B protein that triggers the process of inflammation. Then again, sweet potato is a decent source of fiber, vitamin B 6, vitamin C, complex carbohydrates, and better carotene.

The ingredients help to heal inflammation in your body. These are some of the many foods that are, which can help you in reducing joint pain and arthritis caused by inflammation. Add them to your diet. However, minimize foods that are high in fats, especially trans fats and sugar as they can goad inflammation, joint pain, arthritis, and damage blood vessels, among other related inflammatory conditions.

Rolling out a few improvements will improve numerous things and can have you feeling more energetic and alive than you have in quite a while, and will continue to do as such as long as you remain with the changes you made. This is where many turn out badly. When things have improved, they return to the same old path as before. Try not to sabotage your health; stick with what you are doing, the changes you made, that made you feel better. Try not to return to the old ways what you've done before.

Anti inflammatory diet

CHAPTER THREE
The Anti-Inflammatory Diet - Foods That Heal

What is Inflammation?

Inflammation is a specific procedure with the organic reason to start healing by expanding course. It is a complicated procedure including both the immune system and vascular system and the transaction of different chemical mediators. The extended session brings white platelets and sustenance to the site of damage or disease with the goal that attacking pathogens are executed and harm might be fixed. Trademark indications of inflammation incorporate pain (dolor), heat (calor), swelling (tumor) and redness (rubor).

When Inflammation Goes Awry:

While some inflammation is beneficial and proper for healing, constant or over the top inflammation, filling no need produces harm. Ceaseless inflammation has awful notoriety since it is involved in different disease procedures including (yet not limited to)...

- autoimmune diseases

- arthritis

- diabetes

- Alzheimer's disease

- atherosclerosis (solidifying of veins that prompts heart assault and stroke)

- ADD and ADHD

- sensitivities and asthma

- cancers

- inflammatory gut disease

Delicate tissue swelling and chemical mediators associated with inflammation can likewise disturb nerve endings, adding to the pain.

What is the Anti-Inflammatory Diet?

Different foods are used. Differently, some advancing inflammation and others decreasing it. The reason for the anti-inflammatory diet is to promote ideal health and healing by picking foods that reduce inflammation. If one can effectively control over the top inflammation through natural methods (like through diet), it reduces one's reliance on anti-inflammatory medications that have undesirable and unhealthy reactions and don't take care of the fundamental issue. While anti-inflammatory medicines, (for example, NSAIDs) are a handy solution to ease manifestations, they, at last, debilitate the immune system by harming the gastrointestinal tract which assumes a significant job in resistant system work (1).

Anti-inflammatory Diet Basics:

In general, eat a bounty of fresh vegetables and fruits, entire grains, anti-inflammatory fats, and nuts while limiting prepared foods, meat protein, milk items, refined sugars, artificial hues/flavors/sugars, and food sensitivities.

Vegetables:

Eat and Enjoy:

Enjoy a bounty of fresh vegetables and fruits in an assortment of hues (ideally natural). Fruits and vegetables are much with vitamins, minerals, antioxidants, and fiber, which give the body the fundamental structure hinders for health. Examples incorporate beans, squash, lintels, sweet potatoes, cruciferous vegetables, avocados, dull verdant greens... There are such a large number of decisions! Concerning fruits, pineapple and papaya are especially significant since they are high in bromelain, a fantastic common anti-inflammatory. Fruits and vegetables additionally make great, healthy tidbits.

Avoid/Limit:

Avoid produce that isn't developed naturally. Lethal chemical buildups from herbicides and pesticides can remain and when ingested are remote aggravations to the system. Numerous yields in North America are likewise hereditarily designed and are put available without thorough scientific investigation to decide security for human utilization. Free research is at long last being done to demonstrate the dangerous impacts of devouring hereditarily modified life forms (2). Outside DNA is arbitrarily embedded into the genome of a harvest. Examples incorporate herbicide safe corn and soy, which are impervious to the herbicide Roundup, made by Monsanto.

Generally, 90% of all corn and soy sold in North America is hereditarily modified.

Additionally, know about subsidiaries of hereditarily modified fixings, (for example, corn starch and corn syrup and so on.). It has likewise been recommended that devouring GMOs is a contributing variable to the ascent in hypersensitivities as our bodies are perceiving these food substances as outside (3). By picking things with the "certified natural" name, you avoid both GMOs and dangerous herbicides/pesticides.

For certain people, vegetables in the nightshade family may represent a worry. Examples of nightshade vegetables incorporate tomatoes, peppers, potatoes, and eggplant. Nightshades contain alkaloids which are thought to fuel inflammation and joint harm in certain powerless people with arthritis (however research is clashing). Along these lines, for certain people, limiting or avoiding nightshade vegetables might be beneficial.

Fats:

Eat and Enjoy:

Enjoy healthy, anti-inflammatory fats including olive oil, coconut oil, avocados, nuts, salmon, and sardines. In people, there are two organic fatty acids, alpha-linolenic corrosive (an omega-3) and linoleic corrosive (an omega-6). These are "basic" since they are required for good health; however, the body does not combine them. Omega-3 fats are anti-inflammatory. Omega-6 fats can be professional inflammatory or anti-inflammatory (as it tends to be used by two different pathways). Scientists recommend that keeping the proportion of omega-6 to omega-3 somewhere in the range of 2:1 and 4:1 is best for health. The advanced diet tends to be high in omega-6 as it is richly accessible in cooking oils. Along these lines, including rich wellsprings of omega-3 is significant, (for example, fish, flax and walnuts particularly).

Avoid/Limit:

Fats to limit or avoid incorporate margarine, spread, shortening, hydrogenated oils, trans fats, immersed fats, and milk fat. Omega-6 fats are high in corn oil, safflower oil, and sunflower oil. Trans fats are connected with inflammatory diseases (4).

Meat:

Eat and Enjoy:

In general, limit creature proteins since they tend to acidify the body and furthermore promote inflammation. When choosing creature protein, enjoy fish, poultry (particularly unfenced and naturally raised), sheep and omega-3 eggs.

Avoid/Limit:

Limit hamburger, pork, shellfish, and plant cultivated eggs. In general, grass-fed is better than grain-fed. Avoid hot foods, smoked foods, and cold cuts. Cold cuts contain nitrates and nitrites which promote cancer. Grilled foods contain polycyclic fragrant hydrocarbons (PAHs) and heterocyclic amines (HCAs), which likewise develop cancer.

Dairy:

Eat and Enjoy:

Enjoy dairy substitutes with some restraint, (for example, almond milk).

Avoid/Limit:

Avoid or limit dairy items in general. This incorporates milk, yogurt, cheddar, and dessert. As we age, we lose the catalyst that condensations dairy, bringing about lactose narrow mindedness and inflammation. The milk protein, casein, is additionally acidifying which (in spite of what numerous people are raised reasoning) burglarizes the bones of calcium.

Grains:

Eat and Enjoy:

Enjoy entire grains as opposed to refined grains. Refined grains will be grains in which the germ and wheat have been evacuated. This implies there is a loss of fiber, minerals, and vitamins. In the end, the great stuff is expelled in return for a more drawn out period of usability. Some genuine examples of healthy grains incorporate (natural) entire wheat/oats/ bulgar/couscous, quinoa and whole oats (like steel-cut oats).

Entire grains are likewise a rich wellspring of complex carbohydrates. Complex carbohydrates (as opposed to straightforward sugars) will avoid spikes in your glucose level. Sugar promotes inflammation.

Avoid/Limit:

Avoid or limit refined carbohydrates, for example, white bread, baked goods, sweet things, and pasta.

Nuts:

Eat and Enjoy:

Enjoy nuts and nut spreads, for example, almonds, walnuts, sesame seeds, pumpkin seeds, and flax.

Avoid/Limit:

Avoid a specific nut hypersensitivities.

Drinks:

Eat and Enjoy:

Enjoy a lot of pure, separated water (avoiding chlorine, fluoride, and different contaminants which are aggravations that promote inflammation). Other great decisions are lemon water and homegrown teas.

Avoid/Limit:

Avoid sugary soft drinks, fruit juice (with sugar included) and milk.

Flavors:

Eat and Enjoy:

Numerous characters reduce inflammation. Some great examples are turmeric, oregano, rosemary, ginger, garlic, and cinnamon. Bioflavonoids and polyphenols reduce inflammation and battle free radicals. Cayenne pepper is additionally anti-inflammatory, as it contains capsicum. Capsicum is regularly utilized in pain-alleviation creams.

Sugars:

Eat and Enjoy:

Enjoy stevia, molasses, maple syrup or nectar as better choices for refined sugar.

Avoid/Limit:

Avoid refined sugar, fructose, and particularly high fructose corn syrup which promote inflammation. Avoid artificial sugars.

Other:

Eat and Enjoy:

Enjoy fermented foods, for example, kimchi, miso soup, and sauerkraut. Fermented foods are probiotic and help to revamp the immune system by supporting healthy microflora in the gut and to reduce inflammation. Fermented foods additionally tend to be accessible to process and are likewise production lines for B vitamins.

Avoid/Limit:

In general, kill handled foods, artificial hues, artificial flavors, and additives. Additionally, avoid foods that you have a referred to affectability or allergy to as this promotes inflammation. Poor quality sensitivities are easy to miss, so if you're uncertain, have a food allergy test. Probably the most well-known issue foods incorporate wheat (gluten), corn, soy, milk, and nuts.

All that we require for health can be found in nature. We need to pick well. If you need assistance and thoughts of what to eat, there are a lot of anti-inflammatory diet formula books accessible.

What Else Can You Do to Reduce Inflammation?

- Chiropractic care supports the immune system and reduces inflammation!

- Reduce introduction to natural poisons, (for example, smoke)

- Reduce pressure (5)

- Particular sorts of activity reduce inflammation - specifically, long haul, slowly dynamic preparing, avoiding over-effort (6)

The Fungus Anti-Inflammatory Diet and How it May Treat Your Nail Fungus

What is nail fungus?

By what method may the Anti-Inflammatory Diet Help Treat It?

The anti-inflammatory diet can help support your immune system, which can help fight off parasitic infections. Drinking the prescribed six to eight glasses of water a day is proposed with this diet, which can purify your inward system, likewise fighting off disease.

Notwithstanding being helpful in the fight to free oneself of a fungus infection, there are other health advantages appended to the diet, for example, help with sorrow and improved mental express, a more grounded resistant system, less water retainage, and the sky is the limit from there.

What is the Anti-Inflammatory Diet?

The anti-inflammatory diet, for the most part, comprises of eating 2,000 to 3,000 calories every day. The measure of calories relies upon your size. You ought to eat 40 to half of the sugars, 30 % of fat and incorporate starches, fat, and protein with every dinner.

This diet utilizes a great deal of fish and crisp products of the soil while limiting the utilization of cheap food meals. Beans, winter squashes, and sweet potatoes are additionally a significant piece of this diet.

This diet isn't commonly implied for weight loss, however, can be utilized for health reasons and is said to help with parasitic issues.

How would I know if it's working?

It ought to take a short time for the diet to work. Keep in mind, if you've been eating an entirely unexpected diet, especially if it were a horrible eating routine, it would take some time for your system to be gotten out. You should need to make a visit to a nutritionist or to the neighborhood health food store to examine how and when the diet will work.

You can anticipate that any treatment should take six to twelve weeks to work, and the adjustment in your diet alone may not be sufficient. Write down of what you eat and do and any progressions you check whether you are uncertain of the adequacy of treatment.

Alright, I'm on a diet, what else would it be a good idea for me to do?

Once more, this is something to be talked about with your healthcare doctor, a dietitian or nutritionist, or even your health foot store agent who is knowledgeable in dietary needs. Now and again, a health food store may have different or more dependable data than the web or even your doctor's office and might most likely give you a few enhancements, topical creams or natural enamels which may demonstrate to be incredibly powerful, mainly related to the anti-inflammatory diet.

You may likewise need to check your library or nearby book shop. Web research can be helpful when settling on a choice concerning educational books on nail fungus and diet-related and other natural treatment cures.

An Anti-Inflammatory Diet For Leaky Gut Disease

Leaky gut disease or leaky gut syndrome is a condition that can be caused by antibiotics, infections, parasites, toxins, or terrible eating routine. The significant feature of the situation is alteration or damage to the bowel lining as the coating becomes more permeable than ordinary, it permits microbes, undigested food, waste, toxins, or large macromolecules to enter.

Some researchers believe that these substances have a direct effect on the body; others think the problem is an immune reaction to those substances.

Whatever has caused it for you, you most likely wish the symptoms - everything from acne and indigestion to anxiety and fatigue to joint agony and obstruction, to name a few - would go away. Unfortunately, that desire can lead to treating only the symptoms. If you have Leaky Gut Disease, however, it's significant that you don't merely address the symptoms. You need to concentrate on the root causes of the condition.

One - if not the principal one - of these root causes is diet. While practitioners disagree on a lot of things about Leaky Gut Disease (whether it even really exists, for example), the diet mostly recommended for those suffering from it - the anti-inflammatory diet - is generally acknowledged to be a healthy one for nearly everyone.

The anti-inflammatory diet isn't a diet; it's more of an eating plan. What's more, if you complete a little research, you'll see that there's not only one anti-inflammatory diet; there are several, each with a different turn. For our purposes here, I've tried to present what is a "generic" version. This version does share with the others the concept that continued, and wild aggravation leads to illness and that following an eating plan that abstains from inflaming the body promotes health and can help prevent disease.

In general, an anti-inflammatory diet includes:

- Plenty of foods grown from the ground

- Plenty of whole grains (e.g., dark colored rice, bulgur wheat)

- Lean protein (e.g., chicken, fish)

- Anti-inflammatory spices (e.g., curry, ginger)

- Omega-3 fatty acids, (for example, those found in fish, fish oil supplements, and pecans)

- A reduction in

- Refined carbohydrates (e,g., pasta, white rice)

- Red meat and full-fat dairy foods

- Saturated and trans fats

- No refined or processed foods

Numerous who endorse this diet likewise urge that you dodge refined sugar and items that contain it just as caffeine and liquor. And keeping in mind that drugs don't fall into the diet category, have your specialist review your prescriptions and screen your use of OTC drugs, especially NSAIDs.

One expression of alert regarding this plan: The affects you experience (i.e., an improvement in your symptoms) won't be as immediate as they would be if you treated yourself with medications. You most likely need to give the anti-inflammatory diet, in any event, two weeks versus the hour or two a medicine might take. On the other side, this diet might have a reward effect not generally found in medications: weight misfortune!

10 Tips for Practicing the Anti-Inflammatory Diet

Inflammation and maturing go connected at the hip as inflammation markers - particularly the ESR (erythrocyte sedimentation rate) -

gradually increment with every decade. Many age-related infections have inflammation as their shared factor, and this is incompletely balanced by eating routine, so here are 10 simple tips to stay away from the development of harming inflammation products however much as could be expected:

Skirt the sugar. Diabetes is the traditional model of quickened maturing, and sugar is made of void calories in any case. The drive to devour glucose is inborn, I know, yet pick fresh fruit servings of mixed greens. You will get your sugar fix and a few supplements as an afterthought.

The sweet tooth is the part a great many people find difficult about driving a healthy lifestyle, and most conventional desserts are made of eggs, milk, margarine, and flour which are baked in the appliance. That is the ideal recipe for cutting edge glycation finished results: you have proteins, sugar, and high temperatures. The outcome is the Maillard response. We as of now 'bake' from inside as time cruises by, so why add more glycation? You could attempt crude vegan treats in return. These are made with nuts, seeds, and fruits and don't include any heating or preparing.

Consequently, they are quicker to make too. Recently, crude vegan cake shops have begun to jump up all over. If there is no such spot where you live, look online for homemade vegan dessert recipes, particularly if you have a soft spot for desserts.

Try not to give the multi-day a chance to go without eating a plate of mixed greens and add whatever number different fresh ingredients to it as could be allowed.

Dodge smoked meat and cheese. Same for barbecued meats. In the two cases, you have the troubling blend of high temperatures and proteins which effectively get denatured. The utilization of these kinds of products is connected to stomach related malignant growths in populaces, where they are expended in high amount. There are better approaches to get ready animal products, so why hazard it? You could attempt marinated fish or non-smoked matured cheese. Eat a couple of animal products as could be allowed - once every week ought to be sufficient.

Use the most minimal potential temperatures when cooking. If you are preparing peppers, you could use a lower temperature and a more extended time than if you would bake meat. You would prefer not to eat crude meats and get contaminations. Use your best judgment when cooking.

Use high dampness levels when cooking. It's much improved to bubble and sear than to dish or broil ingredients. If you are an enthusiast of firm food, that would be difficult to execute. Then again, many fresh vegetables and fruits are usually firm if you feel the requirement for it - peppers anybody?

You needn't bother with oil to cook. A fired container/pot and a tad of water will do, and food won't stick. Cleaning is a breeze a while later.

Abstain from heating fats. You can generally add cheese, avocado, nuts, and seeds in your recipes later on. Try not to bake, sear or broil these. The cheese will dissolve in any case if you place it over hot fresh potatoes, and the final product will be similarly as delicious.

Water ought to be your default refreshment. Everything else - soups, teas, and so forth - is a reward and they will never supplant water, regardless of whether the human body will work with what is accessible and it will concentrate water from them. Individuals get progressively got dried out with age at any rate, and numerous substances encourage if you don't drink enough water, so why speed things up when water is so uninhibitedly accessible and shoddy? I surmise if you can peruse this post, at that point access to clean water isn't an issue. Lamentably, that is not the situation for everyone.

Eat as fresh as could be allowed. If you need to eat meat or seafood, get it clean and possibly use solidified ingredients if nothing else is accessible. Try not to cook more food than you eat in one sitting. Heated food isn't as fresh or delicious as promptly set one up. Are you unreasonably occupied for that? I get it, that is the reason fresh vegetables, fruits, and nuts were developed in any case! You could add some quality yogurt and other sound bites when you don't have sufficient energy to cook.

Are any of these 10 hints difficult to actualize? I think not. If you have discovered any use in them or if you have any more tips, remarks or proposals, I'd love to get notification from you! Inflammation and maturing go connected at the hip as inflammation markers - particularly the ESR (erythrocyte sedimentation rate) - gradually increment with every decade. Many age-related infections have inflammation as their shared factor, and this is incompletely balanced by eating routine, so here are 10

95

simple tips to stay away from the development of harming inflammation products however much as could be expected:

Skirt the sugar. Diabetes is the traditional model of quickened maturing, and sugar is made of void calories in any case. The drive to devour glucose is inborn, I know, yet pick fresh fruit servings of mixed greens. You will get your sugar fix and a few supplements as an afterthought.

The sweet tooth is the part a great many people find difficult about driving a healthy lifestyle, and most conventional desserts are made of eggs, milk, margarine, and flour, which are baked in the appliance. That is the ideal recipe for cutting edge glycation finished results: you have proteins, sugar, and high temperatures. The outcome is the Maillard response. We as of now 'bake' from inside as time cruises by, so why add more glycation? You could attempt crude vegan treats in return. These are made with nuts, seeds, and fruits and don't include any heating or preparing.

Consequently, they are quicker to make too. Recently, crude vegan cake shops have begun to jump up all over. If there is no such spot where you live, look online for homemade vegan dessert recipes, particularly if you have a soft spot for desserts.

Try not to give the multi-day a chance to go without eating a plate of mixed greens and add whatever number different fresh ingredients to it as could be allowed.

Dodge smoked meat and cheese. Same for barbecued meats. In the two cases, you have the troubling blend of high temperatures and proteins which effectively get denatured. The utilization of these kinds of products is connected to stomach related malignant growths in populaces, where they are expended in high amount. There are better approaches to get ready animal products, so why hazard it? You could attempt marinated fish or non-smoked matured cheese. Eat as a couple of animal products as could be allowed - once every week ought to be sufficient.

Use the most minimal potential temperatures when cooking. If you are preparing peppers, you could use a lower temperature and a more extended time than if you would bake meat. You would prefer not to eat crude meats and get contaminations. Use your best judgment when cooking.

Use high dampness levels when cooking. It's much improved to bubble and sear than to dish or broil ingredients. If you are an enthusiast of firm food, that would be difficult to execute. Then again, many fresh vegetables and fruits are usually firm if you feel the requirement for it - peppers anybody?

You needn't bother with oil to cook. A fired container/pot and a tad of water will do, and food won't stick. Cleaning is a breeze a while later.

Abstain from heating fats. You can generally add cheese, avocado, nuts, and seeds in your recipes later on. Try not to bake, sear or broil these. The cheese will dissolve in any case if you place it over hot fresh potatoes, and the final product will be similarly as delicious.

Water ought to be your default refreshment. Everything else - soups, teas, and so forth - is a reward and they will never supplant water, regardless of whether the human body will work with what is accessible and it will concentrate water from them. Individuals get progressively got dried out with age at any rate, and numerous substances encourage if you don't drink enough water, so why speed things up when water is so uninhibitedly accessible and shoddy? I surmise if you can peruse this post, at that point access to clean water isn't an issue. Lamentably, that is not the situation for everyone.

Eat as fresh as could be allowed. If you need to eat meat or seafood, get it clean and possibly use solidified ingredients if nothing else is accessible. Try not to cook more food than you eat in one sitting. Heated food isn't as fresh or delicious as promptly set one up. Are you unreasonably occupied for that? I get it, that is the reason fresh vegetables, fruits, and nuts were developed in any case! You could add some quality yogurt and other sound bites when you don't have sufficient energy to cook.

Are any of these 10 hints difficult to actualize? I think not. If you have discovered any use in them or if you have any more tips, remarks or proposals, I'd love to get notification from you!

Master Cleanse Diet Recipe

The master clean diet was created more than sixty years back by an alternative medication expert who made it his central goal to get a safe, productive, and viable route for people to dispose of toxic substances from their bodies alongside assistance in weight control.

Routinely called the "lemonade diet" because of its real fixing, this technique of detox and weight the board has been hip among celebs, particularly individuals who required to lose the pounds rapidly for a film role. Naturally, there are numerous that welcome it since it's a natural, safe approach to get over a night of overwhelming, Hollywood walking. As a general rule, various famous people confess to utilizing the master clean systems to shed weight or tone up their figure. The positive results of the said diet have come on account of the medical advantages of the 3 first master clean fixings. Right off the bat, naturally, there's a lemon, which offers hostile to oxidant control that cleanses the liver and kidneys. This is joined with cayenne pepper, which is a characteristic calming that guides indigestion so clearing the guts.

In the long run, maple syrup, which is wealthy in natural confused sugars just as B-nutrients, gives energy on a cellular level which provides you with more energy without the accident that accompanies many "energy" supplements. While the weight loss and detox are unquestionably the specified results of a Master Cleanse, they aren't the sole advantages. There are a few medical problems that go with these upgrades. For example, inside an underlying couple of days, you may encounter a colon detox and cleaning, as your body begins to separate fat stores and different toxic substances put away in your system. Naturally, over the progression of time, this boosts energy.

Detoxing your system can likewise result in progressively clear skin, better digestion, and general cleaning of your body. This takes into account a bigger supplement osmosis and more energy preservation.

Toward the end, if you pursue the clean master bearings, you may almost certainly shed practically twenty pounds in fourteen days. The master clean diet is recognized every a few months, and although it is commonly used in a non-lasting style, numerous individuals keep on using it till they achieve their general weight loss goal. Bring at the top of the priority list, in any case, that is not safe as a weight-loss program and is saved for accomplishing weight reduction goals.

You should likewise bear as the main priority that since each body is divergent, the results can change. However, these midpoints are decently reliable among the greater part who make progress in the diet plan.

CHAPTER FOUR

Fighting Inflammation One Bite at a Time

Since inflammation is a factor in advancing ailment, it is critical to find a way to kill the inflammatory process. Luckily, nature made numerous things to enable us to fight inflammation. Certain foods have mitigating properties that can reduce the uneasiness of inflammation. Fusing foods that fight inflammation into your present diet will improve your health and help you to feel good. This natural way to deal with inflammation can reduce your reliance on physician endorsed medications and help reduce their symptoms.

On the whole, how about we investigate foods that trigger inflammation. Foods that are seared with trans fats or are made with hydrogenated vegetable oils are enormous supporters of inflammation. Likewise, food that is high in sugar. These incorporate cakes, treats, white flour, white sugar, French fries, and potato chips to give some examples. Reducing sugar admission can cut down inflammation, and it

103

will assist you with cutting calories, which will help with weight reduction and less joint agony. Most processed foods, red meat, and foods high in sugar and processed starches can exacerbate inflammation.

Soaked fats likewise will, in general, add to inflammation. Cut back your immersed excess admission by picking lean cuts of meat, cutting back overabundance excess and picking low-fat dairy items. Arachidonic acid, found in red meats, changes over to genius inflammatory synthetic concoctions. Cured meats, for example, bacon have nitrites, which likewise increment the inflammatory process. Another approach to decrease soaked fat admission is to confine the utilization of red meats.

Being overweight is another issue in the inflammatory process. Fat cells produce inflammatory synthetics in your body. Watch your calorie admission even from the mitigating foods to be examined later in this book.

Presently, for the foods to eat that fight inflammation!

Antioxidants help to fight inflammation by an official to free radicals. The best wellspring of dietary antioxidants is fruits and vegetables. There is no closure to the positive benefit your body gets from eating a diet high in fruits and vegetables. Eating an assortment of fruits and vegetables gives your body the different antioxidants that can cooperate to decrease inflammation. A general guideline is that the more splendidly colored the fruits and vegetables, the higher the cancer prevention agent content. Eating more fruits and vegetables will likewise expand your fiber consumption. Individuals who consume more fiber will, in general, have less inflammation.

1. Pineapple is a decent decision since it contains Bromelain, a chemical that helps separate proteins. For some individuals, it has a similar torment soothing impact to over-the-counter agony prescriptions, similar to NSAIDs, (for example, headache medicine and ibuprofen). Try not to like pineapple...try taking the enhancement Bromelain. Recollect, Bromelain does thin the blood so if you are on remedy blood more slender check with your specialist first.

2. Exploit the splendidly colored berries, for example, strawberries, cranberries, blueberries, blackberries, raspberries,

and red grapes. Use them in smoothies and treats improved with Stevia. Fruits are additionally stuffed with enemies of oxidants. Berries and fruits are high in fiber and low in fat, and their usual sweetness is an extraordinary trade for white processed sugar. Fruits are additionally valuable to individuals with gout as cherry juice, or cherry cases helps the body to wash out the uric acid that has solidified causing torment.

3. Pomegranates have likewise been appeared to help with inflammation. An investigation in the "Diary of Inflammation" in 2008 indicated pomegranate concentrate reduced the creation of synthetic substances that reason inflammation. Drinking around 6 ounces of pomegranate squeeze multi-day is proportional to the portion utilized in the investigation.

Vegetables are another incredible wellspring of nourishment that restrains the inflammatory process. Numerous vegetables have high centralizations of carotenoids, another cancer prevention agent. They additionally have groupings of calcium and nutrient c.

1. Onions and Garlic. These are bulb vegetables that are high in Quercetin, a synthetic that goes about as a characteristic enemy of histamine. Garlic additionally helps to animate your immune system to fight sickness. There are a few different vegetables and fruits that contain Quercetin including dark and green tea, tricks, apples, citrus fruit, broccoli, tomatoes, cherries, raspberries, cranberries and the fruit of the thorny pear desert plant.

2. Spinach is additionally wealthy in carotenoids and Vitamin E. You can get similar benefits from kale, chard, turnip greens and mustard greens.

3. Sweet Potatoes are delectable, low in calories, have no fat, are wealthy in health-boosting minerals, and supply more carotenoids to fight inflammation. All splendidly colored vegetables, for example, winter squash, carrots, red peppers likewise high in carotenoids.

4. Broccoli is high in nutrient C, and calcium and furthermore fights eye inflammation. Softly steam your broccoli to catch a significant portion of its health benefits.

A few spices are useful in fighting inflammation: these incorporate garlic, ginger, turmeric, and hot bean stew peppers. You can take the previously mentioned spices in case of structure; however, it is amusing to try different things with them in different plans. The activity of these spices is fundamentally the same as calming drugs, yet they are more straightforward on the stomach.

1. Turmeric or Curcumin has long been utilized in Asian prescription to treat constant agony and upset stomachs. It can likewise lower blood sugar, blood weight, and cholesterol.

2. Ginger has similar benefits to turmeric to decrease inflammation and has likewise been appeared to ease joint inflammation torment. Ginger can also help when taken for vehicle disorder.

3. Another flavor that can fight inflammation incorporate oregano, basil, cinnamon, parsley, thyme, rosemary. Attempt an assortment of inflammatory reducing spices to receive all the health rewards.

Omega 3 fatty acids are a standout amongst the best inflammation fighters we could utilize. Eating a few servings of fish seven days, for example, cod, sardines, mackerel, fish, and salmon can support the immune system and fight inflammation. Omega 3's can likewise be found in green, verdant vegetables and pecans and almonds. Coconut and flaxseed Oil are additionally incredible wellsprings of omega 3 fatty acids.

Omega-3's assume a job in reducing interminable inflammatory changes in the body and may dull the agony related to ailments, for example, joint pain. They can likewise lessen the danger of coronary illness if taken all the time. If you don't care for fish, you may make a fish oil supplement to receive these health rewards. Fish oil additionally diminishes the blood. It will be ideal if you advise your specialist you are taking fish oil preceding any medical procedures or counsel your specialist before beginning fish oil if on Coumadin or a headache medicine routine.

Different oils that are great to fight inflammation include:

1. Olive Oil contains a characteristic synthetic called oleocanthal which

hinders indistinguishable compounds from mitigating remedy drug. Just premium, additional virgin olive oil contains high enough convergence of this substance to be valuable.

2. Hemp Oil additionally contains Omega 3 fatty acids to reduce inflammation. This is an adaptable oil that can be utilized for cooking or taken by the teaspoonful.

Nuts are another great wellspring of nourishment to fight inflammation.

1. Pecans are wealthy in nutrient E, which helps the immune system and eating them by the bunches or adding them to dishes can avert coronary illness. They are additionally high in Omega 3 fatty acids.

Populaces, which expend the highest measures of choline and betaine have lower plasma C-receptive protein, interleukin-6, and tumor corruption factor. These are generally proportions of inflammation in the body. To benefit from Choline-rich foods incorporate meat liver, chicken liver, eggs, wheat germ, and dried soybeans, in your diet. Betaine-rich foods include wheat grain, wheat germ, spinach, shrimp, and wheat bread.

Start including a portion of the mitigating foods or enhancements into your diet. You will do your cardiovascular system colossal support just as reducing soreness related to exercise. You may see a decrease in skin inflammation, sinusitis, and agonizing joints. You waste size may likewise decrease due to the lower calorie utilization.

How to Build Your Immune System To Fight Viruses

The immune system is known as the most beautiful and complex systems inside the human body. As a holistic nutritionist, I think about the emergency in dis-ease care. In this way, my soul drives me to compose regarding this matter. I'm increasingly obligated to give healthy decisions for change in a world that has achieved scourge dis-ease in pretty much every part of health around the globe. More education, or devotion, as opposed to medicine, is a central point in making better health for a successful life.

It was one of our ancestors who resounded these words hundreds of years back "If individuals let the Government choose what sustenance they eat and what medicines they take, their bodies will before long be in an as sorry state similar to the spirits of the individuals who live under oppression" - Thomas Jefferson.

The immune system is undermined when there is an over the aggregation of toxins and mucus in the body. If the guilty parties are not diminished to ordinary levels, your immune system debilitates expanding your chance for irresistible dis-ease.

Anybody can achieve a significant feeling of prosperity. Fundamentally, you have to get a wealth of holistic nutrition. That is essentially giving your body the ideal admission of supplements enabling it to be healthy and work ideally for you. Holistic nutrition advances your enthusiastic, mental, and physical execution just as parity. Using complete nutrition brings down your rate of an ailment while pushing life span and youth. The medicine for now and what's to come is associated with holistic nutrition.

Out of the host of supplements that have been identified as fundamental for health, nine of them are viewed as the most significant which are your amino acids, magnificent minerals, essential fats, crucial nutrients, predominant starches, fine fiber, pure water, light, and oxygen. Devouring these ideal supplements day by day, your body progressively revamps itself.

Various advantages of structure your immunity with holistic nutrition can be achieved from the least to the best of ideal vitality, clean intestinal tract, improved stomach related power, increased IQ (sharp personality), adjusted cholesterol levels, speed the recuperation time from infections, improved mental clearness and mind-set, focus and rest quality, and progressively significant, security from disease to an all-inclusive healthy life range.

The polarity between customary healthcare model and traditional/modern medicine can be clarified as pursues. Conventional care sees aversion as utilizing education and mindfulness underlining change in conduct to counteract untimely affliction and dis-ease. Modern medicine oversees identification and screening as a strategy for counteractive action. Modern medicine has its focal points, particularly for crisis cases. A customary feeling of health care puts stock in the "land and seed" treatment. In other words, if your body is sufficient, dis-ease doesn't stand a chance. It considers it to be as the "land" and all the disease-causing components as the "seed."

If the land/body is sufficient or for this situation (barren), regardless of how solid the seed (germ), it won't develop, you can persuade your body to be durable to the point that irrespective of what tags along including malignancy your body can ward it off. This is the reason for concentrating on strengthening your immune system is significant. It's critical to ideal health, (counting weight reduction, infection, torment, and related nutritional lacks.)

As a declaration of good health at age 53, in my mid 30's, I mended myself from eager leg disorder and slight joint torment in my grasp. The treatment that I joined in my routine alongside the holistic lifestyle that I live patched me right away. It was a month, or so later I understood that the discomfort I encountered during my month to month cycle never again influenced me right up 'til the present time. By making safeguard strides of purging to decrease toxins from my system, I changed my entire world. Working with a host of diversified networks in carrying positive change to their present health, I talk with an expert on the advantages of holistic nutrition.

This is the same old thing. Numerous extraordinary researchers and visionaries have grasped holistic nutrition. It wasn't until the nineteenth century this methodology was rediscovered. Famous plants were used for mending and relieving dis-eases during our tribal history. After the Cold War increasingly refined, prepared and synthetic loaded sustenance's rose.

It was Edison in the twentieth century who imagine the decree "The specialists of things to come will give no medicine however will show his patients the care of the human edge, in eating regimen and in the reason and counteractive action of disease." Diet and nutrition are connected to health.

Holistic nutrition and being happy to change out of date convictions and personal conduct standards that make strain and stress for all intents and purposes can reinforce your immunity to counteract dis-ease.

There is one just dis-ease which is shaped by a collection of mucus. If the phlegm isn't managed by keeping it decreased to an ordinary level, it debilitates your immune system expanding your chance for infection.

There is no requirement for me to give you therapeutic insights on the scourge of dis-ease. However, I'd like to include that Dr. Emanuel Cheraskin, teacher emeritus at the University of Alabama Medical said "modern medicine is neglecting to give genuine health care, and making a ton of cash out of it. What we call "health care" is genuinely disease care".

Stay away from The Drug Cycle.

Numerous therapeutic drugs, (for example, painkillers or mitigating drugs) smother the body's normal reactions to the fundamental patrons. They act like toxins in the body and can add to a decrease in health as well as reliance.

These drugs treat the manifestation yet not the fundamental reason. At that point, you need another drug to neutralize the side effects. Your body/health starts to winding descending.

Counteractive action Is Better Than Cure.

The host could compare to the trespasser. When battling infections frequently, it is critical to realize what you are managing. In this

116

theatrical world and body, we live in, microorganisms, viruses, organisms, and parasites are found. Strengthening the body, instead of conquering the attacking life form demonstrates a progressively successful technique.

All in all, making these three fundamental strides; without a doubt, help to improve your immunity.

- Step 1 - Administer usually holistic immune structure supplements to control it up.

- Step 2 - Avoid utilizing immune suppressant and depressant drugs without executing a detox a short time later.

- Step 3 - Utilize a detox/purge occasionally to expel toxins from the body.

The "Breath of Life Detox" 30 Day Regeneration equation keeps us robust and healthy. You will discover a variety of stunning advantages from the plans and treatment utilizing "Breath of Life Detox" holistic living methods.

117

Anti Aging Vitamins and Tips

Nowadays, the fight against aging is as intense as the fight against the disease. right from skin products to plastic surgery, there are numerous approaches to reverse indications of aging. After all, nothing is rewarding to see your face covered with wrinkles and blackheads. Even though you cannot prevent cellular aging, you can improve your skin appearance to help you look and feel great. Unfortunately, numerous people are fighting against aging by basically applying the cream on their skin, forgetting that a brilliant skin begins from inside.

A capable enemy of aging treatment consists of skin products yet besides a healthy diet, and most significant regular skin supplements. The skin is the reflection of your internal state, and your inner layer rely on the diet you take what's more, way of life (consistently physical activities, condition, and so forth.). A solid "skin diet" can restore your cells and expands the immovability and brilliance of your skin, including the skin of your face. Alongside cancer prevention agent cream, it is essential to take cell reinforcement supplements to fight free radicals, which cause a variety of biological effects on the skin. Besides, cell reinforcement supplement help reduce hazard factors for cardiovascular disease, cancer, hypertension, obesity, diabetes, and then some. It is likewise recommended to eliminate in your diet foods high in fat; alcohol and tobacco, which age skin cells, making you look old.

You need to increase the accompanying supplement in your diet:

Vitamin E - advantages of Vitamin E on your skin are tremendous. It battles free radical, advances wounds mending, secures the cell membrane from damage, and helps your skin look younger. Vitamin E participates in the prevention of development or oxidation of cholesterol in your blood; and in particular, it helps in the prevention of numerous diseases that plague our society: heart disease, cancer, cataracts, Alzheimer's disease. Besides, vitamin E underpins healthy immune system.

Sources: Wheat germ oil, sunflower, hazelnut, soy, and corn are wealthy in nutrient E.

Vitamin A - it protects and beautifies the skin. Vitamin A likewise strengthens the mucous membranes (bronchi, veins, and heart). As beta-carotene, it seems to participate in the prevention of certain cancers in non-smokers. Nevertheless, Vitamin An is best when taken alongside vitamin E. foods that contain Vitamin An include liver, butter, egg, carrot, tomato, spinach, apricots, papaya, celery, melon, grapefruit, broccoli, etc.

Note: If you are a smoker, you should contact your physician before you take beta-carotene supplements.

Vitamin C - this basic supplement is the foe of free radicals and disease. Regardless of whether taken inside or remotely, nutrient C anticipates wrinkles and lights up the standard color, texture, and appearance of the skin. Besides, alongside a healthy lifestyle and diet, Vitamin C intervenes in the prevention of lung diseases, stomach disease, and cataracts. Vitamin C is found bounteously in lemon, lime, tomato, parsley, pepper, guava, sorrel, tarragon, kiwi, cabbage, papaya, citrus, strawberry, broccoli, peas, and the sky is the limit from there.

Healthy fats - if you need to have beautiful skin and prevent cardiovascular disease, increase your omega 3 intakes. Omega-3 unsaturated fat likewise relieves severe and incendiary conditions: joint inflammation, prostatitis, cystitis, etc. Besides, this unsaturated fat improves memory function and concentration; make you feel happier, and relieves manifestations and bipolar depression and psychosis. Omega 3 seems to assume a major role in preventing the development of breast, colon, and prostate issues. Fish oil and flax oil are rich in omega-3.

Zinc - if you need your skin to be brilliant, increase (14 mg max) your zinc intake. It assumes a major role in numerous biological functions: development, respiration, endocrine system, healthy irritation response, wound healing, reproduction, and healthy immune system. It seems to participate in the prevention of cancer of esophagus, bronchi, and prostate. Zinc is copiously found in beef, bread, wheat germ, soybeans, white beans, and lentil.

Selenium - Although it is toxic in large doses, selenium supports the immune system, neutralizes poisons, eliminates or counteracts the effects of heavy metals (lead, mercury), promotes the production of sperm and more significantly, prevents premature aging. Associated with vitamin E, it regulates cholesterol and reduces the danger of cardiovascular problems. The accompanying foods are rich in selenium: fish, egg, meat, cheese, barley, garlic, asparagus, broccoli, and orange.

Anti-Inflammatory Cream For Pain Management

You might be comfortable with several brands offering anti-inflammatory creams. The more significant part of these brands has been in the market for a considerable long time. Numerous among these creams neglect to provide the ideal outcomes to the people utilizing it. These creams are vital to the aficionado and athletes of the game.

These creams can offer transient help to the people utilizing it. If pain is persevering for an all-encompassing period, consulting a doctor is suggested. Each brand of inflammatory cream will give you a period after which you should go to the doctor.

Anti-inflammatory creams are ordinarily used for reducing the inflammation in the sensitive body parts. This is especially powerful for the injuries that happen because of overworking.

The essential capacity of the cream is to help the muscles in reducing the pain and inflammation related to overdoing. Other generally used strategies for managing the inflammations are rest, ice, pressure, and rise for diminishing the inflammation. The confronted paced society of today has been a significant reason for every one of these issues. The natural solutions for treating this circumstance are additionally well known. The conventional ways incorporate eating a lot of vegetables, fish, and exceptionally hued natural products. Sustenance things that have the low substance of trans and saturated fat will help you in keeping away from inflammation.

The causes of inflammation are many. The significant reasons are overworking of the muscles that are not implied for working hard, wounds, and so on. A few illnesses like Arthritis and Carpal Tunnel Syndrome can likewise cause inflammation. Attempting an anti-inflammatory cream before heading off to the costly procedures of restoring the inflammations is something worth being thankful for to do.

A large portion of these creams utilize incredible chemicals, and that is the reason why the use of these creams in high quantities and delayed periods are not viewed as useful for the general health of the individual. The admonitions in the jugs of these creams ought to be intently pursued with the goal that you don't need to confront the outcomes. There is a decent plausibility that the chemicals present in the creams can go overdose. The overdose of chemicals like Methyl Salicylate in these creams can be exceptionally hurtful to the users. Use of various cured cushions and creams are regularly found in the athletes. This can cause genuine health problems.

Understanding the home cures accessible for treating inflammation will likewise be useful. The use of regular things like ginger, green tea and so on that will be there in your kitchen can help you enormously in disposing of inflammation. Vitamin E, vitamin C, and omega3 unsaturated fats are among the substances that have an incredible task to carry out in treating inflammation. Notwithstanding, the key lies in utilizing them in the endorsed quantities. Consulting a doctor before taking the prescriptions is the best thing to do. As the number of people, using the anti-inflammatory creams is on the ascent, the people encountering health problems identified with an overdose of the chemicals are likewise expanding.

Anti-Inflammatory Drugs - Fatal Side Effects For Arthritis Sufferers?

Non-Steroidal Anti-Inflammatory Drugs - NSAIDs - are among the world's most broadly recommended drugs, and the most every now and again obtained over the counter (OTC) medicines. They treat pain and as indicated by pharmaceutical industry gauges, around one-fourth of the whole total populace experiences moderate to the constant severe pain.

NSAIDs are drugs containing anti-inflammatory and pain-relieving ingredients that help calm inflammation, fever, and pain. Since inflammation is one of the central causes of pain, the quest for compelling anti-inflammatory operators has been extraordinary. Headache medicine was the primary monetarily significant NSAID, however since it, just the same as different NSAIDs, can aggravate the stomach coating and causing inner dying, the drug companies started the quest for a superior arrangement.

NSAID and Pain

When tissue cells are harmed - for instance, by joint inflammation - inflammation is made and the enzyme, PLA (phospholipase), is discharged. The PLA enzyme separates the external layer, of the harmed cell, yet of neighboring cells. These cell dividers are made of unsaturated fats called phospholipids - which at that point break free.

The separated unsaturated fats are then handled by three further enzymes called COX 1, COX 2, and LIPOX.

The final product of the procedure is the making of another unsaturated fat called a prostaglandin, which is perceived by pain receptors on nerve endings and transmitted to the cerebrum as pain.

Prostaglandins additionally aggravate the first inflammation which makes an endless loop - because more PLA is made and, in this manner, more cell layers breakdown and hence more phospholipids are discharged, and this way more prostaglandin is created. The circle proceeds.

NSAIDs work by keeping the separated phospholipids from coming to COX1 or COX2

- which is the reason they are called COX Inhibitors. Be that as it may, they can't obstruct the pathway to LIPOX.

Besides, they influence the side effects - the pain - they don't address the cause. Furthermore, they can be a cause for gastric ulceration, evaluated to affect the same number of as 20% of NAISD long haul clients.

Undoubtedly the US encounters around 7,600 NSAID-related passings and 76,000 NSAID-related emergency clinic affirmations every year. As indicated by one research bunch NSAIDS cause upwards of 40 crossings for every week in the UK.

Given the genuine symptom issues, researchers started to search for better NSAID's and in the '70s found there were two types of COX, assigned COX-1 and COX-2. It ended up evident that restraining COX-1 was the cause of the ulceration issue, and drug companies started to scan for aggravates that blocked COX-2 without influencing COX-1.

This increasingly specific (enchantment shot) approach, it was trusted, would create a more secure item. It, in the end, delivered the COX-2 inhibitors Celebrex (sold via Searle and Pfizer), Vioxx (sold by Merck and Co.), and Bextra (sold by Pfizer). Security was to demonstrate slipperily.

COX-2 Inhibitors and Cardiovascular Disease

There was doubt very early that COX-2 inhibitors could expand blood pressure. In 2005 this was affirmed by an exceptionally colossal meta-investigation, (an examination of 19 separate investigations of the impacts of COX-2 inhibitors), distributed in the Archives of Internal Medicine. This paper inferred that they did for sure tend to raise blood pressure - a realized risk factor for heart assaults and strokes.

In parallel with this examination, a group at the University Of Pennsylvania School Of Medicine (Zhang '03, Rudic '05) had pretty much settled how the COX-2 inhibitors made this issue. COX-2 has more than one job in the body. COX-2 is engaged with the blend of substances that cause pain and inflammation; yet it is likewise in charge of creating a sleek material called prostacyclin - a heavy atom.

Prostacyclin controls how blood vessels adjust to stresses, for example, hypertension. By decreasing degrees of prostacyclin, the COX-2 inhibitors increment blood pressure. Be that as it may, they likewise quicken the procedure of atherosclerosis (solidifying of the courses), meddle with principal recuperating instruments, and perhaps increment the risk of blood clusters.

This 'flawless tempest' blend of impacts, the scientists proposed, could all cooperate to build the risk of heart assault and stroke even in already reliable people.

Fighting Pain with Nutritional Food Ingredients

Since quite a while ago disregarded by the drug companies, many driving researchers have, in any case, examined the remedial intensity of natural food ingredients and their dynamic constituents. The best-recorded anti-inflammatory is the food flavor turmeric, which has a long history of utilization in Ayurvedic medicine in the treatment of painful conditions from sore throats to joint pain.

The curcuminoids in turmeric lessen pain and inflammation by restraining COX-1 and COX-2, or more the other inflammatory enzyme is known as lipoxygenase or LIPOX. They are amazing antioxidants that lower LDL (the 'terrible') cholesterol and ensure against oxidation. They lessen blood pressure and make the blood less inclined to clump.

Curcuminoids have a place with a more extensive class of phytonutrients called 'flavonoids,' a group of mixes which happen in many plant foods, for example, berry products of the soil are related with better wellbeing prospects - including a lower risk of Alzheimer's.

CHAPTER FIVE

The Anti Inflammatory in Natural Foods

Inflammatory and anti-inflammatory arthritis, these are the most well-known types of joint inflammation. What's the distinction? Fiery joint pain is normally known as rheumatoid joint pain, where the non-incendiary joint inflammation is best known as osteoarthritis. It is regularly the situation that a similar joint inflammation that causes arthritis may likewise be related to other medical issues. Inflammatory arthritis is an inflammatory malady condition coming about because of degeneration of ligament in the joints, causing pain. Rheumatoid arthritis is an auto-invulnerable ailment in which the body's insusceptible system attacks joints, tissues, and organs. A natural process which has an organic reason to help to mend by expanding the course is known as inflammation. It is a process which includes the vascular system and resistant system. This additionally provides an interchange of different compound go-betweens and is known as a complicated process.

Here, the sustenance and the white platelets made by expanded dissemination to the spot of contamination or damage so the attacking pathogens being evacuated and the harmed ones fixed. The qualities of inflammation are heat, redness, swelling, and pain. Inflammation is either treated by meds or the natural route by being on a specific eating regimen. Medications have very little to offer without symptoms or the utilization of pain executioners, so natural calming foods been expended for better execution with no hazard. Be that as it may, different foods being used differently, some of them advance inflammation while others evacuate it.

Picking Anti Inflammatory Foods!

Here is a portion of the mitigating natural foods. Vegetables and products of brilliant green hues help the advancement of inflammatory. Vegetables and natural products are rich in minerals, fiber, vitamins, and cancer prevention agents by which the body gets the basic structure obstructs for wellbeing, for example, squash, sweet potatoes, avocados, beans, lentils, dim green verdant vegetables, and cruciferous vegetables. There are numerous cancer prevention agents and phytochemicals present in the vegetables and natural products that have calming properties. Fats: Foods likel, nuts, sardines, salmon, olive oil, coconut oi and avocados are natural calming foods which are sound. Omega 3 unsaturated fats are likewise physical and inflammatory specialists which change into prostaglandins, a hormone-like substance. The body itself can't make omega 3, this most significant unsaturated fat and like this should originate from the food you eat. These are found in oily fish of virus water like mackerel, herring, and salmon. Too they are found in flaxseed which is otherwise called linseed and its oil. The omega 6 fats additionally help in reducing the pain and inflammation, and these are found in sesame seed oil, safflower, sunflower, and pumpkin. In any case, the omega 6 admission ought to dependably be not as much as omega 3, this proportion is significant.

Flavors That Fight Inflammation!

There are numerous flavors which help in reducing inflammation of which turmeric is the best. It is known as the best calming food for any individual who is experiencing arthritis. Its be either be taken as a supplement or be added to the food in its natural brilliant yellow powder structure. For snappier and better ingestion into the circulation system, it makes it with some dark pepper. Different flavors utilized fin bring down the inflammation are rosemary, cinnamon, garlic, ginger, and oregano. Polyphenols and bioflavonoids, which are found in all the food referenced above, are additionally found in red wine and dim chocolate and can be utilized to decrease inflammation, also fending off free radicals. Cayenne pepper is also calming as it has capsicum present in it and capsicums are regularly used in creams for pain alleviation.

About Grains!

The entire grains are natural calming foods which are rich in complex carbohydrates. The complex carbohydrates help in forestalling spikes in sugar level of the blood, and the sugar advances inflammation. However, one of the pivotal focuses here is, if the grain is refined as it has wheat and germ, through the refining process, there is lost minerals, vitamins, and

134

fiber. Probably the best grains are bulgar, oats, whole oats, quinoa, whole wheat, and couscous. Taking supplements is of an extraordinary advantage since it fills the spot of a portion of the foods you will be unable to eat. When taking supplements, you should comprehend what to make and use demonstrated quality items. A considerable lot of the gels and creams are not the issue solvers. Just by eating the right food and including a decent natural supplement will give you that outcome you were searching for and progressed toward becoming sans pain.

Anti-Inflammatory - A Must Know To Avoid Rheumatoid Arthritis

Inflammation is inside of our body's immune reaction. Without inflammation, at that point, the body will be not able to mend. Arthritis is primarily an "acidic" condition, identified with the inflammation and pain that typifies this disease. The most common structure is osteoarthritis; this comes from a moderate degeneration of cartilage, which is the cushion tissue that lines the joints. Joints primarily affected by arthritis are the knee, hips, fingers, and the vertebrae of the spine.

This type of sickness is frequently confused with osteoporosis, which is another genuine medical problem that affects the bones. Osteoporosis is when your bones become delicate and fragile, losing minerals such as calcium quicker than the body can replace them. This prompts low bone thickness and great danger of fractures. To treat this type of sickness would be entirely different for treating rheumatoid arthritis. With rheumatoid arthritis, there is some genetic tendency. Never the less, there are things you can do to postpone the beginning and limit the indications of this disease.

The first and most significant advance is decreasing acid-framing food. Ther should be a changing your eating routine, exercise may be the exact opposite thing you consider or have a craving for doing. Physical activity improves adaptability, stance, and balance, fabricates muscle, helps bone thickness, facilitates joint-pain and stiffness. Intend to exercise only direct, make sure to go slowly and gradually develop your quality.

When things gain out of power!

Some inflammation is part of the immune system; however, when inflammation is wild, as in rheumatoid arthritis, this will harm the body. Inflammation has a noteworthy influence on diseases such as heart disease, cancer, and weight. Foods rich in trans fats and sugars invigorate swelling, redness, warmth, and pain of the body. They induce over-activity of the immune system. Indeed, even immersed fats in this case, which are useful for the body, be kept at the lower level.

There have been no successful cures with medication for rheumatoid arthritis. Painkillers are frequently used to cope with the indications. Taking an excessive number of painkillers over quite a while is creating numerous different genuine medical problems and be more savage than the disease itself. For overseeing arthritis and joint pain find out about the arthritis type affecting you to assume responsibility for your condition. Examine lifestyle and diet changes, likewise physical activities for pain alleviation and natural enhancements that can help.

Foods That Are Anti Inflammatory

Entire grains are part of anti-inflammatory foods. Eating your grains, whole grains as compared to refined cereals, rice, bread, and pasta helps in reducing inflammation. This is because of entire grains groups a high fiber content. Being high in strands helps bring down the measure of C-reactive protein. C-reactive protein is a noteworthy cause of blood inflammation. Increase antacid shaping foods, such as products of the soil that can be included in a day by day menu. A major increase in alkalinity can come by drinking a green juice day by day, sourced from organic products, veggies, herbs, spinach, parsley, celery, beetroot tops, and wheatgrass.

The same number of studies have demonstrated the inherent anti-inflammatory potential comes from omega 3 fatty acids. Having fish, in any event, three to four servings for each week such as mackerel, salmon, sardines, and fish have a high content in omega 3 fatty acids. These fatty acids are a standout amongst the ideal courses in reducing inflammation. The fish be either bubbled or heated instead of dried, browned or salted fish. You ought to stay away from foods with a high content of omega 6 fatty acids such as fish oil supplements and processed vegetable oils, which can increase inflammation. Vegetable oil sounds solid by name, however, has nothing characteristic and best be maintained a strategic distance from altogether.

Soy: None processed soy products are part of anti-inflammatory foods. They contain estrogens and isoflavones compounds, which help your body in bringing down inflammation levels. You should be maintaining a strategic distance from soy that is vigorously processed. This is because intensely processed supplements in soy pair with additives and added substances, which reduces the supplements contained in regular soy.

Beets: Beetroot and beetroot-juice have nutrient C and plant colors known as betalains that protect against cancer and reduce inflammation. It is additionally realized that the nitrate content of beetroot juice is the way to bringing down pulse, along these lines cutting the danger of heart disease and stroke.

Garlic and onions: Garlic works correspondingly to NSAID medications for pain. It closes off pathways promoting inflammation. Onions have comparative chemicals, including allicin compounds that help in making free radical battling acids.

Garlic, we need it consistently; it is valuable in the counteractive action and treatment of heart disease and enables lower to blood fats, cholesterol, and circulatory strain. There is likewise a fundamental fixing in garlic more dominant than the most two essential antibiotics at battling one of the leading causes of food harming.

Nuts are a decent source of sound fats, in particular, almond nuts, which are rich in nutrient E and calcium, and walnuts, which are rich in alpha-linolenic acid. Nuts have numerous things, such as minerals, calcium, magnesium, and potassium. Together with a low sodium consumption, the minerals are crucial to bone wellbeing. Not just that, they likewise protect against blood vessel hypertension, insulin resistance, and cardiovascular disease.

There is no preferred option for anti-inflammatory foods. These foods guarantee a sound, disease-free life. If you are allergic to the foods referenced than it is fitting to keep away from them for, they may cause increased inflammation.

Anti-Inflammatory DietThat Fight Inflammation Without Drugs

When your body sends a message! Inflammation, in simple terms, is our body's method for advising us that there is something incorrectly. This could be because there are pathogens or even some boosts already in our bodies. Ideally, this helps our bodies to get better. However, if our bodies react, exciting on existing inflammation, a simple bothering end up with swelling and creating discharge. This could be bothering and agonizing, especially as joint pain. Other than the use of medications, foods that are anti-inflammatory help manage inflammation. In assuming responsibility for any health issues, there are some significant focuses to consider. Everything comes back to knowledge; knowing what to do, a fundamental understanding of knowing where to begin and how to go about it.

Where a great many people are turning out badly or are feeling the loss of that critical point is "persistence". Most give up before the benefits begin to work. You should remember, this isn't like a medication that stops the manifestation very quickly, and that is everything it does. A drug doesn't fix the illness itself from whichever part of your body or organ this is originating from. The body will fix it when it gets the correct nutrients, and that is your responsibility.

First Thing First!

Other than anti-inflammatory foods, one should watch their body weight. Keeping up the correct weight for your height is a more common way to deal with battle numerous health issues incorporating inflammation, for example, on account of joint pain. Studies have likewise demonstrated that exercise is a significant part to help fight inflammation. This mostly needs gentle exercise. For instance, Yoga goes far in reducing interleukin-6, which is an inflammatory marker. Whichever part of the body has the problem, gentle movements, stretching exercises in the shower or shower will help. The secret is to combine these things, for example, diet, the correct sustenance, minerals, vitamins, exercise, and every one of them applied like team-work will have the best outcome and a positive result. Any of those used individually in attempting to fix a problem will have little or no effect.

Anti Inflammatory Foods!

Obscure to a great many people, there are healthy foods you may eat under typical circumstances, and yet they can increase inflammation. Thus, let's take a gander at the food that is anti-inflammatory and will help to manage inflammation. Adding to your diet, for example, olive oil, avocado oil, or even grapeseed oil will enable you to get your meal's nutrients faster. These oils go well in servings of mixed greens and make it taste great. These are some of the oils that are great in reducing inflammation as they contain mixes, for example, oleic acid, which is an omega-9 unsaturated fat that helps your body to fight off inflammation. Eating fish instead of beef additionally helps in eliminating inflammation. Meat has more salt and cholesterol, which is a major no-no when dealing with inflammation. It is significantly changing to anti-inflammatory foods, for example, fish. Fish has an abnormal state of omega-3 unsaturated fat, which fends off inflammation and is an excellent source of protein. This includes fish like fish and bass. Maintain a strategic distance from farmed fish if possible. Chicken ought to likewise be part of the diet as it is leaner than beef.

The fiber in Your Diet

Increasing your fiber intake likewise helps to reduce inflammation and expending whole grains, which are a decent source of foods that are anti-inflammatory instead of refined grain items that, for the most part, have added sugar. This keeps the C-reactive protein under control. Instead of refined sugars, increase organic products in your diet by eating a few between meals. These include pineapples, apples, strawberries, and practically any natural product you extravagant, and they likewise go well with nuts, for example, pecans and almonds. They increase the omega-3 fat, alpha-linolenic acid, and vitamin E. These types of unsaturated fats are less likely to give a heart assault. Alpha-linolenic (ALA) is part of omega-3 and especially significant in the diet because our body can't make it sans preparation.

To improve your diet, likewise, increase the measure of green vegetables you eat. Vegetables like kale and spinach have abnormal amounts of vitamin E to fight off inflammatory, causing molecules. They likewise beneficial because of its calcium and iron, which are necessary minerals your body needs. Discuss great-tasting cures, and you are discussing chocolate. Chocolate with no less than 70% cocoa falls under the anti-inflammatory food types, has less harmful fats, and would be an excellent method for fighting inflammation.

To put it plainly, keep off foods that are not anti-inflammatory, for example, those containing added sugars or/and saturated fats, as these increase inflammation in your body. If despite everything you think this is more like an invalid's meal and lacking taste, well reconsider. Including garlic, ginger, and delicious herbs, for example, oregano, bean stew, parsley, thyme, and spices, turmeric can add that extra taste to pretty much anything. The end-result and the most significant benefit: they all have been proven to fight inflammation better than all else with no side effects.

Natural ANTI-INFLAMMATORY Diet For Better Health And Less Pain

Inflammation is perceived by pain, swelling, redness, and warmth around the influenced zone. There are different choices to treat inflammation. One is meds, which so far hasn't been best since it doesn't generally fix the issue. The other alternative is a natural way, from where our body begins from; our body been made commonly and gets its unique items from nature. This implies choosing the food that your body needs since setbacks of secure fixings doubtlessly caused the disease in any case. It is likewise comprehended our body can respond differently to foods since certain foods being used separately to other people. What that implies, as in inflammation, a few foods can have a positive or a negative outcome. Here are a portion of the common calming foods; if chose accurately, they will make that difference in mending.

Normal Anti-Inflammatory Foods

Vegetables and organic products: Vegetables and products of green and splendid shading help the procedure of fiery conditions. Vegetables and natural products are rich in antioxidants, for example, vitamins, minerals, fiber which the body needs each day to remain healthy. There are numerous assortments, per model, squash, sweet potatoes, avocados, beans, lentils, dull green verdant vegetables, and cruciferous vegetables. These have multiple antioxidants, phytochemicals, and calming properties present.

Important Fats

Additionally, rich in calming foods are olive oil, coconut oil, salmon, sardines, and avocados. Every one of them contains omega 3 unsaturated fats which are fundamental for inflammation and joint health. The corrosive from omega 3 is a fiery specialist that changes into prostaglandins, which is a hormone-like substance. Omega 3 isn't useful for joint pain and inflammation. It is likewise essential for health when all is said in done. We can get omega from our diet, in this manner it is necessary to incorporate a portion of the healthy oils such as olive, coconut, macadamia, and krill, which is more grounded than fish oil. There are numerous choices of foods accessible which contain a variety of omega.

Oils you should think about

Olive oil has more health benefits than a great many people figure it out. Make sure to utilize it in your diet; however much as could reasonably be expected. Olive oil is great in antioxidants and is containing a substance called oleuropein. Therapeutic science has established that additional virgin olive oil is one of the healthiest foods we can add to our diet. This oil is most useful and powerful for joint inflammation sufferers since it can cool inflammation and straightforwardness joint pain. Be that as it may, for cooking, singing, heating and so forth utilize just coconut or macadamia nut oil. Different oils when warmed become poisonous and as a rule transform into trans-fats which can trigger inflammation and joint pain, only as other health issues. Keep away from these oils: Vegetable oils, soybean, canola, these are the more typical ones a great many people think about on account of the names. Indeed, they have the right sounding name, yet they are not healthy.

Flavors

Turmeric would be over the rundown in reducing inflammation and joint pain. Also, turmeric has compound curcumin, which is known for some, health benefits and can fix joint pain. It is best utilized in its typical fine structure and added to your diet when conceivable, the more, the better. Other prominent flavors used for reducing inflammation are cinnamon, rosemary, garlic, ginger, and oregano. This is great in polyphenols and bioflavonoids which help to lessen inflammation just as ward off free radicals. Cayenne pepper is likewise known for its mitigating property and its capsicum content which is added to certain creams for pain relief.

Grain

Entire grains which contain starches can likewise help in forestalling spikes in the sugar level of the blood, as it is realized that sugar advances inflammation. Be that as it may utilize just not refined entire grains, when preparing has occurred all the decency is lost, for example, vitamins, minerals, and fiber. Among the best grains are oats: Whole oats, entire wheat, quinoa, couscous, and Bulgar. To take a multi supplement is of advantage, it can fill the spot of certain foods you generally may not get from your diet as required day by day. Be that as it may, your first need should dependably be the diet, just then when taking an enhancement, you will get best worth.

Make It Work!

The correct kind of food and supplementation is essential to treat joint inflammation, inflammation, and joint pain. Multivitamins that contain vitamin C, E, zinc, B 6, copper, and boron are a great idea to have incorporated into your diet. It has been discovered that a few

149

supplements inadequacy in patients could be the reason for experiencing joint inflammation. There is likewise solid proof that exercise is similarly as crucial as your diet. Anybody enduring joint inflammation pain, the exact opposite thing you would consider is exercise. You abstain from moving as meager as conceivable because each time you move, it makes pain. Exercise is the choice to joint pain relief since it breaks the propensity to support your joints and to maintain a strategic distance from the development. Shirking of growth and exercise will, at last, make the pain more regrettable and debilitates the body.

Few out of every odd diet has a similar impact on each one. When choosing a specific diet, the vast majority have not the tolerance to proceed and to attempt a variety of things. Inflammation and joint pain are certifiably not a convenient solution; it will require some investment and persistence. I have voyaged this street recognizing what's included. I likewise realize it is reachable with consistency. When you began don't surrender.

Who Should Eat the Anti-Inflammatory Diet?

Did you realize that inflammation has been identified as the reason for most endless disease - diseases like arthritis, weight, diabetes, heart disease, and much malignant growth? Truth is stranger than fiction. Most perpetual conditions are a consequence of a lifestyle of prosperity that manages us the advantage of having the option to eat the off-base foods in the off-base amounts at the off-base occasions. These food choices set in play a large group of procedures in your body that produce inflammation from a considerable number of sources. Furthermore, a significant amount of us are hereditarily customized to provide over the top inflammation when presented to regular aggravation sources, for example, smoke, synthetics, and poor dietary choices. A few of us produce so much inflammation that we have autoimmune disorders, for example, lupus, multiple sclerosis, rheumatoid arthritis, psoriasis, and colitis.

How precisely do poor food choices produce inflammation? Bundled and exceedingly prepared foods just as fast foods are a portion of the most noticeably terrible guilty parties.

151

They are additionally a portion of the food choices most generally accessible. Intended for accommodation, these foods are stacked with trans-fat to broaden their timeframe of realistic usability just as change their taste and surface. A trans-fat is made from an essential, saturated fat - another not exactly healthy fat. This saturated fat is "transformed" into a trans-fat using a procedure called trans-hydrogenation. This transformed fat is synthetically different enough from an essential fat that, when fused into your body tissues, it makes a course of synthetics called cytokines. Cytokines are molecules in charge of creating inflammation all through your body.

Foods that are stacked with refined sugars are additionally inflammatory. Cakes treat, and doughnuts are instances of foods that are quickly processed by your body, discharging a lot of glucose. This glucose is consumed rapidly by your body, causing a high blood glucose level. Your body this way releases a flood of insulin to help standardize your blood glucose levels. This flood of insulin joined with high blood glucose levels makes your body discharge cytokines, inflammatory molecules, too. Each flood of glucose flags your body to store fat. Prepare to have your mind blown. Fat tissue turns out to be physiologically dynamic and starts to discharge these equivalent inflammatory molecules, cytokines, too.

Refined grains - grains deprived of fiber and crucial supplements likewise make inflammation. An entire grain is a molecule made out of a lot of glucose connected and embodied with a fiber coating. This fiber coating makes the absorption and arrival of glucose a gradual procedure. When the external fiber coating is stripped away to make a smooth and rich surface, glucose molecules are promptly accessible for fast assimilation and retention into your body. This quick flood of glucose into your framework again is the trigger for the inflammatory course.

Individual grains can produce inflammation in specific people. Wheat, oats, grain, and rye are on the whole grains that contain significant amounts of a protein substance called gluten. Gluten makes foods, similar to bread, crunchy outwardly, and delicate within. However, this equivalent gluten is exceptionally inflammatory in people hereditarily tested in processing gluten. Indications can be as extreme as pain, swelling, the runs and ailing health or as gentle as sickness or absence of vitality. Taking out these specific grains from your diet is frequently the way to controlling this sort of inflammation.

What precisely is an anti-inflammatory diet? All in all, an anti-inflammatory diet comprises of fresh, entire foods which don't contain triggers for inflammation and are stacked with molecules that neutralize inflammation in your body.

Phytonutrients are found in many products of the soil, in charge of their vivid appearance. These large molecules have antioxidant just as anti-inflammatory properties. This implies they neutralize the oxidative pressure that your body produces day by day, prompting inflammation. Healthy fats found in chilly water, fatty fish, flaxseed, and nuts can likewise lessen the amount of inflammation produced by your body also. Cooking oils, for example, olive oil and canola oil additionally help your body battle and neutralize inflammation. Certain nutrients and minerals - nutrient A, D, E, and C, just like zinc, selenium, and copper - are found in wealth in new, entire foods. These antioxidants likewise neutralize oxidative pressure and hose the arrangement of inflammation.

Wiping out fast foods just as bundled foods is the initial step of the anti-inflammatory diet. Killing foods with refined sugars and handled grains is the subsequent step. Eating liberal amounts day by day of crisp leafy foods and moderate amounts of entire grains and lean protein just as healthy fats found in fish, seeds, and nuts are the foundation of the anti-inflammatory diet. At that point for select people, diminishing or taking out grains, particularly gluten-containing grains, is the last step.

So exactly who ought to eat an anti-inflammatory diet? Any individual who experiences an inflammatory condition, for example, autoimmune disorders (lupus, multiple sclerosis, rheumatoid arthritis, colitis.) or unfavorably susceptible disorders (asthma, dermatitis) will profit by the anti-inflammatory diet. A great many people with dull pain (migraines, back pain, neck pain, knee pain, joint pains, nerve pains, muscle pains) have components of inflammation engaged with their pain and will profit as well. Fractious inside disorder and essential stomach related disorders, for example, indigestion improve with the anti-inflammatory diet. However, shockingly, anybody enduring constant degenerative diseases (arthritis, diabetes, heart disease, and much malignancy) will also profit from this diet. At last, anybody keens on counteracting these neurodegenerative diseases and accomplishing ideal wellbeing will benefit. The science affirms that eating to forestall inflammation averts disease and keeps up wellbeing as well as keeps us looking and feeling more youthful.

So, eat healthily and don't give the inflammation a chance to get it together on you. From kids to the old, everybody can profit by this ground-breaking way to deal with eating.

CONCLUSION

Joint pain is challenging to live with and can seriously influence your daily life. Arthritis and some other type of joint pain can make even the most straightforward development difficult in your ordinary day's exercises. You may feel like taking a pain pill to ease the pain rapidly. These calming prescriptions have opposite side effects and delayed utilization of these pills can really make lasting harm a portion of your body organs and furthermore the safe framework. Rather than picking to use over the counter prescription, there is a superior and more secure strategy like including natural calming nourishment in your daily diet, which has constructive outcomes to your health.

Although a not insignificant rundown of natural fruits or vegetables ends up overpowering to a few, yet there are different alternatives accessible. Items with equalization, assortment, balance, health disapproved of the blend of all the common fruits including the Acai berry, too omega-3 for its most calming effect are accessible in a fluid enhancement. Taking these two times each day makes it a simple path for your body to get every one of the fruits and benefits.

Notwithstanding, underneath are a portion of the six significant mitigating regular fruits that can help ease arthritis joint pain, and inflammation and the sky is the limit from there.

1. Pineapple!

Besides having an incredible taste, pineapple is a well-known common mitigating fruit. The fruit has a compound called bromelain, which helps in reducing inflammation as well as helps in reducing the pain and supports the recuperating procedure. Truth be told numerous arthritis medications use pineapple concentrate to treat the condition. If you are experiencing joint pain, eat new pineapples, and you will feel the difference. Maintain a strategic distance from canned pineapples since they contain some additional sugar and additives which can have the contrary effect and are not suitable for your health.

2. Berries!

A wide range of berries, including strawberries, blueberries, and raspberries are extraordinary mitigating fruits. They contain cell reinforcements as well as all the significant

158

phytochemicals which soothe the joints and furthermore evacuate poisons that are destructive for the body. You can eat them entire or in a type of Smoothies to ease the joint pain. These berries are likewise wealthy in nutrient C, which helps arthritis and ligament pain.

3. Papaya!

This isn't just a delectable fruit yet besides, an incredible specialist that can ease pain and inflammation. It has a catalyst considered papain and different minerals and vitamins that help to calm soreness and throbs. Papaya likewise helps to advance healthy hair; it is right for your skin and furthermore helps in processing. They are natural calming fruits that are profoundly prescribed by nutritionists in light of other health benefits.

4. Bananas!

Bananas are a good wellspring of numerous vitamins and minerals which help fortify joints and battle arthritis. There are numerous other amazing motivations to eat bananas. Here are some healthful realities of bananas: Vitamin-B6-5mg, Manganese-3mg, Vitamin-C-9mg,

Potassium-450mg, Dietary fiber-3g, Protein-1g, Magnesium-34mg, Folate-25.0 mcg. For these numerous health reasons and benefits, bananas are a significant fruit to add to your daily diet.

5. Cherry!

Research has demonstrated that cherry juice can decrease joint pain, and it is as per Eve Campanella, Ph. D. She came to locate that the majority of her patient's accomplished joint pain alleviation in the wake of drinking a glass of cherry juice two times every day.

6. Apples!

Squeezed apple and fruit purée all have calming properties which can prevent and fix arthritis and different types of joint pain.

Taking everything into account, mitigating natural fruits are significant because they make you healthy as well as assistance to prevent and fix joint pain and arthritis, which has turned into a typical issue to numerous individuals. There is likewise a point to recollect, cures like this work slower than medication prescription; however, have no side effects and will give you proceeded with health.

Here is a little treat for you by the day's end. Have and appreciate a glass of red wine with your supper; ensure it is dry, for example, Cabernet, Merlot, or Shiraz and so forth. One to two glasses of dry red wine every day will give you the conventional benefits of the cancer prevention agents and resveratrol in red wine. The ingredients of red wine bring down your LDL cholesterol as well as too bring down your circulatory strain. It additionally reduces inflammation in your body. Recollect, two glasses are sufficient; that sum even keeps your stomach related framework healthy too.